THE END OF FOOD ALLERGY

THE **END** OF
FOOD
ALLERGY

The First Program to
Prevent and Reverse
a 21st-Century Epidemic

KARI NADEAU, MD, PHD

Director, Sean N. Parker Center for Allergy and
Asthma Research at Stanford University

AND **SLOAN BARNETT**

New York Times Bestselling Author

AVERY
an imprint of Penguin Random House
New York

AVERY

an imprint of Penguin Random House LLC
penguinrandomhouse.com

Most Avery books are available at special quantity discounts for bulk purchase
for sales promotions, premiums, fund-raising, and educational needs. Special
books or book excerpts also can be created to fit specific needs. For details,
write SpecialMarkets@penguinrandomhouse.com.

Library of Congress Cataloging-in-Publication Data

Names: Nadeau, Kari, author. | Barnett, Sloan, author.
Title: The end of food allergy: the first program to prevent and reverse a
21st-century epidemic / Kari Nadeau, MD, PhD, Director, Sean N. Parker
Center for Allergy and Asthma Research at Stanford University, and Sloan
Barnett, New York Times Bestselling author.
Description: New York: Avery, Penguin Random House, 2020. |
Includes bibliographical references and index.
Identifiers: LCCN 2019055419 (print) | LCCN 2019055420 (ebook) |
ISBN 9780593189511 (hardcover) | ISBN 9780593189528 (ebook)
Subjects: LCSH: Food allergy—Prevention. | Food allergy in
children. | Immunotherapy.
Classification: LCC RC596 .N33 2020 (print) | LCC RC596 (ebook) |
DDC 616.97/5—dc23
LC record available at https://lccn.loc.gov/2019055419
LC ebook record available at https://lccn.loc.gov/2019055420

Printed in the United States of America
10 9 8 7 6 5 4 3 2 1

Book design by Lorie Pagnozzi

To the patients—the true heroes of our story

CONTENTS

THE **END** OF **FOOD ALLERGY**

Part I

UNDERSTANDING FOOD ALLERGY

Chapter 1

INTRODUCING *THE END OF FOOD ALLERGY*

Who we are, why we're here,
and what's ahead

Welcome to the future of food allergy.

If you're reading this book, then you're probably affected by food allergy in some way. Or maybe you're simply interested in understanding more about this epidemic gripping the country and, increasingly, the world. Perhaps your baby was just diagnosed with an allergy to nuts or dairy or egg. Maybe you have a child in elementary school confined to the nut-free table in the cafeteria and you're turning down invitations to birthday parties out of fear that an accidental exposure to wheat or dairy will send him or her to the hospital. Maybe you have friends with food allergy in their family or their own diagnosis. Maybe you are a clinician wishing you had more options for your patients. Or maybe you're a parent anxious about putting your food-allergic child into anyone's care but your own.

It could be that you're a teacher with food-allergic children in the classroom. Or maybe you have a teenage family member who seems always on the verge of forgetting to bring their epinephrine when they go out with friends. Or maybe you are the one in your family who has never tasted peanut, the result of arranging your life around avoiding places and foods where your allergen is likely to lurk.

3

Whoever you are, if you are one of the tens of millions of people touched by food allergy in some way or are simply curious about the condition, then this book is for you. This book is here to help.

Food allergy is entering a new era. For decades we have grappled with this alarming and perplexing epidemic that has affected an increasing number of children and adults. Yet science has had little to offer to those fated to a life of fear about possible death (albeit very rare) by accidental exposure.

That time is over. Gone are the days when avoiding a food at all costs was the only option, when nothing could be done and no one had any clues about treatment. We are also done with the years when claims of food allergy were met with skepticism, ignorance, and dismissal. Both science and the general public now recognize this condition as a serious disease that requires our help.

For the past century, food allergy researchers have been forging a new continent. Hard-won understandings about the immune system now form fertile ground that allowed something new to grow: options.

Immunotherapy is at the heart of this new world. This powerful technique trains the immune system to stop treating a given food as an enemy. It sets the body back on course by reeducating it, slowly but surely, about the safety of nuts or wheat or eggs or dairy, or whatever other food triggers the dangerous, self-harming reaction known as an allergy attack.

EXPLORING A NEW LAND

This book provides an in-depth look at the complete program for preventing, diagnosing, and reversing food allergy. Part One starts with the harrowing numbers showing the dramatic rise of the condition over the past thirty years or so. We unpack the various theories seeking to explain this increase in prevalence, collecting the grains of truth scattered across this field of research. Next we address one of the most pernicious side effects of food allergy: parental guilt. We look at what the science tells us about pregnancy diets, breastfeeding diets, genetic inheritance, and other possible pathways through which food confusion may enter the immune system. With self-blame set aside, we then tackle the kitchen, guiding families on everything they need to know about changes to make at home following an allergy diagnosis—including a clear-eyed walk through the tangled mire of food labeling laws.

Part Two delves into the heart of the new era for food allergy. It begins with a look back at how we became so focused on avoidance as the only option. Equipped with the lessons of the past, we then shift to knowledge we now have about preventing food allergy. We make a clean escape from the avoidance myth aided by rigorous research on early introduction. And we offer an evidence-based, practical guide for when and how to add new foods into our diets in order to prevent food allergy.

That brings us to immunotherapy. To put it simply: it is now possible to treat and reverse food allergy. The research is still in progress and we are still identifying standard regimens that allergists everywhere can offer in their clinics. But the thousands of patients who now live free from the fear of accidental exposure—many of whom freely eat their former allergens as if they never had a bad reaction to them—are a testament to the power of this program. The new era for food allergy is all about returning control to people's lives. Immunotherapy is one way that happens.

We include information to help you decide if immunotherapy is for you, how you can become a study participant or be treated safely in a clinic, and what other cautions you will need to take into consideration as you step into this new era. In short, we equip you with all you need to know about this new treatment. We give you a map of the landscape, tell you how to get around, show you the best sights, and make sure you have a place to stay.

But there is so much more to this new moment for food allergy. Research and development pipelines are full of products, from new medications to wearables to (of course) apps. We look at every corner where advances are now under way, with a dose of healthy skepticism. This view of the not-too-distant future is a realistic one, focused on what might truly assist you and recognizing that the money to be made from the food allergy "market"—that is, people living with the condition—is reason for caution.

In the final section, we address an aspect of food allergy that has been under-recognized for far too long: the emotional toll. We look at the research showing just how much the condition affects all members of a family, and offer plenty of wisdom, for children and parents, about how to cope. The voices of teenagers and young adults who grew up with food allergy and now live on the other side provide invaluable insights.

Finally we consider our part in the future health of the planet. The rise of allergy is not separate from many other dire issues we are confronting. And so the suggestions in the last section are aimed at not only preventing food allergy but also reducing our impact on the earth. The new era of food allergy rests upon the truth that we do not have to accept the status quo. Our choices make a difference.

ABOUT YOUR GUIDES

Before we go any further, we want to share our own stories. For both of us, our initial connection to allergy was personal. But spreading the word that a new time has begun has become a mission. Our goal with this book is to tell you everything we know so that you can make informed decisions for yourself and your family. We'll start with telling you about us.

Kari

My career in science and medicine has been dedicated to the care of children and adults suffering from food allergy. In the clinic and in the laboratory, I study the immune system and work with collaborators around the world who share the vision of preventing and treating food allergy.

My first exposure to the world of allergies arrived as a toddler growing up in New Jersey. My father, a marine biologist, was researching how pollution affected the water and marine life. Part of that work meant studying animal life at the bottom of a river—which meant living on a houseboat. A moldy houseboat. And it turned out that I was terribly allergic. Between that and my bad asthma, I gained an early appreciation of just how much our surroundings can affect our bodies.

Working as an emergency medical technician when I was 16—the ambulance was the first car I ever drove—helped me realize I wanted to be a doctor. I joined one of the first freshman classes to include women at Haverford College. Thanks to a scholarship and the excellent teachers there, I had my first glimpse of molecular biology and the profound inner workings of our cells, including the immune cells responsible for allergies. I decided to pursue both research and medical care, earning my MD/PhD at Harvard Medical School through the Medical Scientist Training Program, sponsored by the National Institutes of Health (that program also introduced me to my future husband).

One day in 2003, when I was a clinical trainee, my mentor and I were called to the intensive care unit. I was a fellow in asthma, allergy, and immunology by then, learning under Dale Umetsu at Stanford University. I followed Dale to the ICU, where a father approached us in tears. He held a plastic bag containing an epinephrine autoinjector. I could see the needle was bent. "I don't understand," he told us, "I don't understand."

But very soon Dale and I understood the matter all too clearly. The father's 9-year-old son had been diagnosed with a milk allergy when he was a toddler. Doctors at the time knew very little about milk allergy, and the family was left with the impression that it would fade. One night, their son accidentally drank from his sister's glass of milk. When allergic symptoms appeared, his family tried the epinephrine, but the dose was sized for a small child. He went into anaphylactic shock and within twelve hours his brain had swelled so much that there was no hope of saving his life.

The story didn't end there. The child became a liver donor and the recipient developed a milk allergy. I had little clue about why that would happen and was determined to find out by studying the immune system. And I knew I wanted to do something to stop completely preventable deaths like this one. I could see that researching the mechanisms behind food allergy and finding ways to improve the care of people living with the condition were inseparable aims. For me, they became inseparable dreams.

As I delved further into the world of food allergy, parents and patients started approaching me. We met in cafés around the world, where they shared the struggles they had with their children's allergies or their own. As family after family asked if there would ever be a way to do something better for people with food allergy, I resolved to help them. These conversations evolved into extensive involvement with the food allergy community. This community has been invaluable in guiding my work by pointing me toward the most pressing needs and questions. Other allergy centers were having good results with experimental approaches to treating milk, egg, and peanut allergy. Within a few years, my team at Stanford was conducting the first-ever clinical trial of immunotherapy combined with the asthma drug omalizumab, which blocks a crucial component in severe reactions, for the treatment of milk allergy. The study included just eleven patients, but the results amazed us. Several patients could tolerate a much higher amount of milk within nine months; for some, the change took just three months. That success was repeated in our next study, this time treating people with more than one food allergy.

I met Sloan and her family in 2013, when she approached me about treating her children for their allergies. In the years that followed, we spoke often about finding a way to tell others about the revolutionary transformation happening with food allergy. Her vision, compassion, and sheer drive led us to create this book together. As the research progressed, I wanted to ensure that families and patients would know all they can about preventing and treating food allergy, and so did she—which led to the book you now hold.

Sloan

I was plunged into the world of food allergy at a restaurant near our home in New York when my son was 2 years old. He started to seem sick and we figured he was coming down with a cold. But when I put him into bed at home, I realized his heart was racing. My husband and I rushed him to the nearest emergency room, and after two days in intensive care, he was diagnosed with asthma. The doctor told us that our son would need to be tested for food allergy because it's so common among children with asthma. When he was diagnosed with peanut allergy, the doctor then suggested that our daughter, who was just 6 months old at the time, be checked, too. She tested positive for tree nut allergy. The experience was entirely new for me. I remembered that the captain of the squash team at my college had died from an allergic reaction to peanuts. But no one in my family had ever encountered a threat like that.

My family relocated to California when my children were 4 and 5. Allergy attacks seemed to follow our daughter around the world. Wherever she went, some kind of tree nut residue seemed to find her. We managed to keep peanuts away from my son entirely, but I saw the threat of food allergy up close, again and again, as my daughter grew up.

Then one day at a wedding, a couple seated at our table began talking about their own experience with a food-allergic child. "You live near Kari Nadeau," they told us. "Haven't you met her?"

I hadn't—and decided to remedy that fact right away. It turned out that the timing was perfect. My son enrolled in a trial investigating a new treatment for peanut allergy and my daughter enrolled in one for tree nut allergy. For the next year, I made the ninety-minute drive to Stanford every week so one child or the other could have their treatment dose increased. It was never easy, but the possibility of overcoming this potentially fatal condition made the challenge worthwhile. And the incredible bedside manner upheld by Kari and her team made us confident that we were in the safest hands possible.

Later, when my children had both overcome their allergies and

Kari and I had become friends, I encouraged Kari to bring this work to the world. I could see what a brilliant researcher and physician she was, and believed her prodigious gifts deserved a wider audience. By then, Kari knew about my background as a lawyer, a journalist, and author of the bestselling book *Green Goes With Everything,* a guide for clean and healthy living. She knew that I was just as passionate as she was about broadening environmental awareness, identifying the causes of food allergy, and spreading information about treatment options to as many people as possible. So we joined as coauthors to help families everywhere access the knowledge and feel empowered to steer their own ship. Our vision for the future is simple: the end of food allergy.

Both

For ease of reading, we refer to ourselves throughout the book as "we." Sometimes, "we" is also used for Kari and her research team. Anything pertaining to clinical trials at Stanford University comes directly from Kari's experience. All the patients mentioned in this book agreed to share their stories here. All of the approaches taken by patients and families in this book were based on their personal decisions. We urge any parents or newly diagnosed adults to consult with professionals about any interventions they take in preventing or treating food allergy.

A FUTURE BUILT BY MANY HANDS

Scientific progress is the very definition of a joint effort. We move forward incrementally, one study at a time, building off one another's findings. We talk about our results, we meet at conferences, we keep each other encouraged, and quite often, we become friends.

The new era of food allergy was brought into existence by the many dedicated researchers and physicians who persisted with their work over decades, and continue to do so today. They recognized that food allergy was a serious condition worthy of countless hours in the laboratory and hard-to-come-by research dollars. And they never let go of the idea of finding a treatment. They even dared to dream of preventing and curing food allergy. The work of these researchers and physicians is included throughout this book, and we are glad to bring their pioneering discoveries together in this way. We apologize for any inadvertent omission of important and intriguing food allergy research currently under way or that has brought us to where we are now.

This book also draws on our research at Stanford University and our experience caring for patients and their families, whether during clinical trials or as part of routine allergy management. We are honored to include insights from the patients, parents, researchers, clinicians, and children who are directly impacted by food allergy in this book.

PREPARING FOR THE JOURNEY

The science of food allergy is an ongoing, worldwide effort. Researchers are attempting to understand incredibly minute and detailed processes of the immune system: the interaction of our immune system with the environment; the role of genes in shaping the inner workings of immunity; the outer influence of our surroundings; the proteins in various foods and our body's handling of them; the effect of different types of drugs on all of this; and so much more. All of which is to say: this story is hardly finished. Rather, it's just beginning. And that means we don't always have a firm conclusion, a definite answer, a consistent result. Some studies contradict one another. Some findings can be interpreted in different ways. And new findings are emerging all the time, which means we need to be flexible in our thinking. What seems true today may not seem that way a year from now, given the pace of the research.

We don't sugarcoat the research and we don't shy away from presenting studies that give opposing results. We believe that equipping people with information means presenting as complete a picture as we can. It is typical (and necessary) for scientists to harbor healthy skepticism about new research. After new data and their analyses are adequately discussed and repeated, facts can emerge. To that end, we have presented a summary of facts in our "bottom line" comments. And we give you our promise that each of these is based on the best evidence available today.

And while we are on the subject of science—there's a lot of it. The future of food allergy is based on research, and we want you to know the discoveries that decades of research have produced. We also want to ensure that anyone touched by food allergy feels at ease navigating the data. We hope you will talk to board-certified allergists. Those discussions and the knowledge gained from this book will equip you to draw your own conclusions about what the evidence means for your life.

Every study we've included in this book is there because it is part of the story. It's fine to breeze through the study descriptions quickly and focus more on the summaries. You will still leave this book with a clear sense of what the new era of food allergy is all about. If you take the time to consider each of the investigations, then you will have a deeper understanding of the history of food research and you will understand how science has wrestled this new approach into existence. Either way, we encourage you to not feel intimidated or confused by the science and the numbers. They are here to serve you, not the other way around.

The End of Food Allergy includes a full list of all the studies we've referred to throughout the book. A hyperlinked version of the list is available at TheEndOfFoodAllergy.com. We also include a glossary and three appendices. The first contains a list of organizations and networks where food allergy families can find support of all kinds. The second appendix is a concise debunking of common myths about food allergy. The third is a disclosure listing all financial ties between ourselves along with anyone interviewed for this book and any for-profit companies involved in food allergy treatment and prevention. We want all of you reaching for this book to feel confident that the information you are receiving is unbiased and based squarely and solely on our best evidence to date. Our singular driving motive is to ensure that anyone who wants knowledge about the current best ways to address food allergy can have it.

FOR THE NEWLY DIAGNOSED ADULTS IN THE ROOM

Developing a food allergy as an adult is more common than many people think. Although much of the public discourse on food allergy focuses on children, the population of people diagnosed with food allergy when they are over age 18 is growing. More than 10 percent of American adults are allergic to at least one food. Nearly half of this population developed at least one food allergy as an adult. For nearly a quarter, adulthood was the first time they'd ever experienced the condition. The situation is similar worldwide.

Almost all of the information in this book applies to everyone with food allergy, regardless of age. Clearly, adults living with this condition don't need to worry about keeping risky snacks out of reach in the pantry or handling the nut-free table in the cafeteria. But nearly everything else is universal. Although the language in this book is often directed toward parents of newly diagnosed children, adults with food allergy can read this as applying to them equally. It will be obvious where the information is specifically for children.

Most important, the groundbreaking treatments presented here are for people of all ages. Many food-allergic adults have successfully completed immunotherapy and now live free from the fear of encountering their former allergen. The new era of food allergy is life-changing for everyone.

SPEAKING THE LANGUAGE

Finally, it will help to know some basic terminology. Certain words are often used interchangeably or unclearly in the world of food allergy. So we want to make sure that the specific meanings of words used frequently throughout this book are clear. We also include a glossary at the back of the book with more definitions.

Allergy: The hives, itchy skin, wheezing, watery and itchy eyes, nasal congestion, coughing, mucus, and low blood pressure that the body produces when it encounters a food that the immune system incorrectly identifies as harmful. This reaction involves a type of immune cell called immunoglobulin E, or IgE for short. Allergy research often uses the term *IgE-mediated allergy* to indicate a specific immune-guided reaction, which is different from having a food sensitivity that triggers, say, temporary gastrointestinal discomfort.

Desensitization: Treatment interventions that increase the amount of an allergen that a person is able to take without having an allergic reaction are known as desensitizing treatments. Desensitization is the overall process of increasing the "dose" of allergen over time.

Intolerance: The phrase *food intolerance* is different from *food allergy*. An intolerance might cause bloating (such as from lactose) or a headache (such as from MSG). Some people experience rashes from certain spices and fruits (such as cinnamon or pineapple). When a person says, "I can't eat beans, they make me gassy," or "I can't eat peppers, they bother my digestive system," they are referring to an intolerance that is not life-threatening.

Sensitivity: Some people have food sensitivities that cause discomfort, sometimes serious discomfort, but these, too, are not a food allergy for the purposes of this book. With celiac disease, a person may have severe diarrhea after eating wheat. That's a serious condition that needs to be considered by restaurants and processed food manufacturers, but it isn't a food allergy by definition. Also, a person may have some amount of IgE directed against a particular food without actually being allergic; this scenario also comes under the umbrella of sensitivity rather than food allergy.

Tolerance: Tolerance refers to the body's not reacting against a protein, whether it comes from inside the body (insulin, for example) or outside (peanut, egg, or milk, for example). Most of us are naturally tolerant of all foods. Sometimes tolerance arrives soon after the first or second year of life, a common scenario with egg allergy. Therapy-induced tolerance means the immune system is trained out of a food allergy or other reaction (such as rejection of a donated organ). In this state, the person does not need constant exposure (say, one peanut a day) in order to maintain tolerance. In the field of food allergy, we now refer to this state as *sustained unresponsiveness*. It's too soon for us to say whether the retrained immune system will stay that way for the rest of a person's life—in other words, whether that person is cured. There are now individuals who have remained tolerant even after a full year of not consuming the allergen. A result we once dreamed of is now a reality. Sustained unresponsiveness is the closest we come to saying a person is cured—for now.

One final note: Throughout the book, any mention of egg allergy refers to hen's eggs and any mention of milk allergy refers to cow's milk.

Chapter 2

THE FOOD ALLERGY EPIDEMIC: WHAT IS HAPPENING—AND WHY

What we know and don't know about the causes behind the staggering numbers

Natalie Giorgi had always been careful. Diagnosed with peanut allergy at 3 years old, she had to be. Avoiding the legume (peanuts are actually not nuts at all) had become one of her earliest life skills. Like many children, she developed a "Spidey sense" that knew when her enemy, the peanut, was near.

Then came the summer of 2013 and her family's fourth annual trip to a camp in the woods near Lake Tahoe. Prompted by emails and phone calls from Natalie's parents each year, the camp made sure to keep the food peanut-free, and their prior vacations had been without incident. Which is why Natalie thought the Rice Krispies Treats she'd eaten on previous visits to the camp were safe to eat.

After one bite, Natalie, who was 13 at the time, knew something was different. She ran to her parents and told them she thought she might have eaten peanut butter. They gave her Benadryl and waited. Nothing happened. Had they been wrong about her allergy all these years? Had she outgrown it?

A few minutes later she vomited. Her airway began to close. Her father injected her with epinephrine and then gave her a second dose, then a third, but the reaction was unstoppable. The ambulance took a long time to arrive because of the remoteness of their location. By the time Natalie reached a hospital, doctors couldn't save her. She died that night from a single bite of a Rice Krispies Treat made with peanut butter.

THE NUMBERS

Natalie was hardly alone in the threat she faced. By all reports, food allergy among children has risen steeply in recent years and is continuing to do so. Adult-onset food allergy is also increasing.

Tallying just how many children in the United States are currently living under the kind of threat that Natalie faced is tricky. The only way to know for sure if children have a food allergy is to give them the food and wait to see if they react. But most of the studies measuring the prevalence of food allergy rely on questionnaires completed by parents, with no guarantee of how the condition was diagnosed. Some parents may mistake digestive issues, headaches, or symptoms caused by a food not agreeing with a person for one reason or another for an allergy. A survey seeking to find the rate of food allergy—that is, the percentage of children in a given population— may overestimate the statistic because parents of food-allergic children are more likely to participate (a phenomenon statisticians call selection bias). Some allergy tests have a high rate of false positives, confirming the presence of an allergy where none exists, again leading to inflated estimates. The rate of egg allergy depends on whether the eggs used to test for a reaction are raw or cooked. All these variables can make it hard to grasp the nationwide and worldwide prevalence.

And yet even with all of these factors taken into account, the statistics are clear: food allergies have skyrocketed in the past couple of decades. One of our main sources for that assertion is the federal collection of studies known as the National Health and Nutrition Examination Survey (NHANES). According to the most recent NHANES survey, between 2007 and 2010, 6.5 percent of U.S. children were living with food allergy. That's nearly 5 million children, or 7 out of every 100. A more recent study by researchers at Northwestern University, led by Ruchi Gupta, puts food allergy prevalence at 7.6 percent of U.S. children. As for adults, a 2014 estimate put the prevalence among U.S. adults at about 5 percent, or about 14 million. A 2019 survey that we conducted with researchers at Northwestern of more than 40,000 U.S. adults found that nearly 4,400—11 percent—had food allergy. Applying that figure to the U.S. population as a whole means that more than 26 million U.S. adults harbor an allergy to peanuts, shellfish, dairy, or other food. And out of every 100 patients with food allergies, about 6 will be allergic to just one food but 40 will be allergic to at least two, often more. Regardless of whether you focus on the most or least conservative figures, it's clear that food allergy is rampant in the United States.

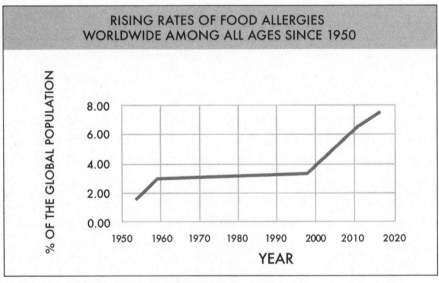

RISING RATES OF FOOD ALLERGIES
WORLDWIDE AMONG ALL AGES SINCE 1950

BASED ON DATA FROM MULTIPLE PEER-REVIEWED SOURCES.

That's also true around the world. In 2013, an international group of researchers led by the World Allergy Organization reported food allergy rates as high as 15 percent among the 89 countries included. According to their findings, food allergy is not a phenomenon

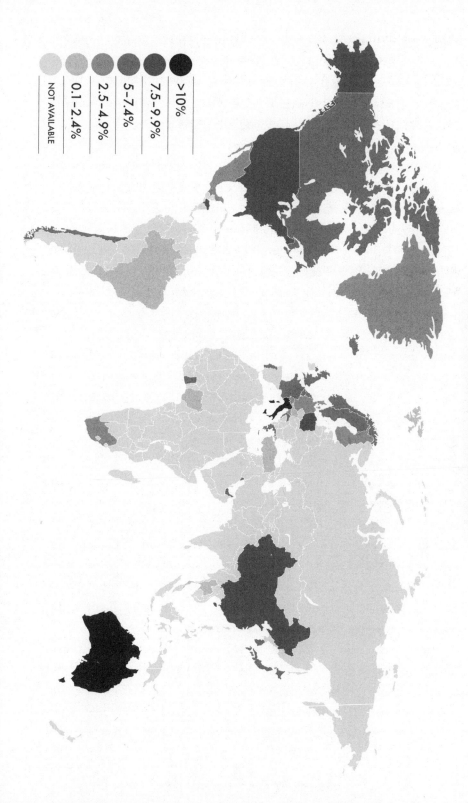

GLOBAL PREVALENCE OF FOOD ALLERGY

>10%
7.5-9.9%
5-7.4%
2.5-4.9%
0.1-2.4%
NOT AVAILABLE

unique to Western countries. Australia, Finland, and Canada top the charts for children age 5 years or younger; Mozambique, Tanzania, and Iceland have the highest rates for older children. Taking all children, from birth to age 18, the UK, Colombia, and Finland rank as the top three. In other words, food allergy is a global phenomenon that is only becoming worse.

It wasn't always like this. The shift has been well documented since the late 1990s, and some researchers trace it back to the 1950s. According to the Centers for Disease Control and Prevention (CDC), food allergy prevalence among children increased 3.4 percent between 1997 and 1999. Between 2009 and 2011, it increased another 5.1 percent. These percentages may seem small, but we look at them in a real-world context: that's more than an additional 1 million children with food allergies in less than fifteen years. Hospital visits for food allergy increased threefold from 1993 to 2006. Again, the United States isn't alone. In China, for example, food allergy among infants increased from 3.5 percent in 1999 to 7.7 percent in 2009. In the early 1990s, 16 out of every 1 million children were admitted to hospitals for food allergies in the UK annually. By 2003, that number had climbed to 107 out of every 1 million.

Peanut allergy is especially rampant. Back in 1997, less than half a percent of U.S. children were allergic to peanuts. By 2008, the rate had climbed to 1.4 percent. Over the next seven years, prevalence nearly doubled, bringing the rate to 2.2 percent by 2018. Dairy may be even worse. In one 2007 survey, 17 percent of respondents reported milk allergy. All of the eight most common food allergens—eggs, fish, crustacean shellfish, tree nuts (almonds, hazelnuts, walnuts, pistachios, and all others), wheat, soy, along with milk and peanuts—have seen increased rates in recent years.

Race and ethnicity matter. A 2016 study of 817 U.S. children from Chicago, Illinois, and Cincinnati, Ohio, found that asthma and eczema (known risk factors for food allergy) were more common among African American children than among Hispanic and white children. Compared with non-Hispanic white children, African Amer-

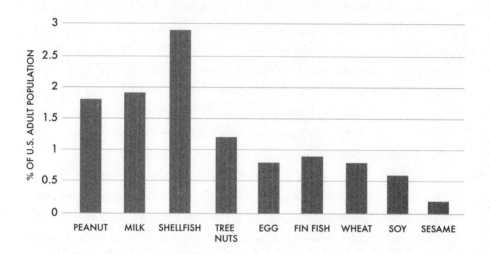

THE NINE MOST COMMON FOOD ALLERGENS AMONG U.S. ADULTS

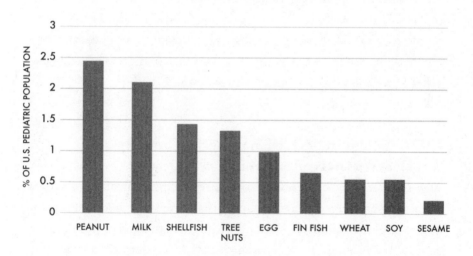

THE NINE MOST COMMON FOOD ALLERGENS AMONG U.S. CHILDREN

ican children were also at high risk of allergies to wheat, corn, soy, fish, and shellfish. Hispanic children had more instances of allergies to corn, fish, and shellfish compared to white children in the study. Currently food allergy rates are highest among non-Hispanic black children. Studies have found higher rates of shrimp allergy among non-Hispanic blacks compared to non-Hispanic whites. Other research showed that black children are more likely to be allergic to several foods at once. And a study looking at food allergy trends between 1997 and 2007 reported the most significant increase among Hispanic children. "African ancestry was a notable risk factor for increased risk of peanut sensitization," notes one summary of the data. Researchers have a long way to go toward understanding how and why ethnicity plays a role in food allergy, and how to address this risk factor effectively.

Geography also factors into food allergy risk. Where a person lives may influence the foods they're allergic to—mustard seed allergy is particularly common in France, for example, and royal jelly allergy relatively more common in Hong Kong. The exact immune mechanisms behind a food allergy sometimes differ among countries. The peanut protein that people react to in one country may be different from the protein that people react to in another. Although the majority of food allergy research has been conducted in Western countries, the worldwide prevalence is increasing (we address these numbers in chapter 11). Countries where the condition was once unheard of are now struggling to address its rise.

THE HYGIENE HYPOTHESIS—WHAT'S RIGHT, WHAT'S WRONG, AND WHAT'S NEXT

The numbers can be dizzying and overwhelming, but they carry a clear message: something is happening across the world. Food allergy is a global epidemic. Which leads to the question of why. What's going on? What has changed in the last few decades that has left our bodies so confused about what foods are safe to eat?

Science has generated valuable insights and a wealth of data about the mechanisms behind food allergy. Some of this work has seeped into mainstream knowledge, leaving allergy sufferers with vague ideas and theories based on legitimate but limited research. The hygiene hypothesis is probably the most well-known explanation behind food allergy and other immune disorders. Which means this is a great opportunity to unpack this theory, in all its fact-based and not-so-fact-based glory.

This term may be familiar to many readers, and the hypothesis, though overhyped, may explain some portion of the food allergy epidemic. The theory is all about immunity. When we're in the womb, our immune systems are virtually a blank slate—and rightfully so. This system is geared in part to reject foreign substances, but a growing fetus has to be open to receiving whatever the mother sends through. And we don't need to be on guard when we have our mother's antibodies to protect us. After birth, that situation changes. Outside the protective womb, a baby has to learn to protect itself. It has to station its own sentries to guard the castle and send out soldiers when invaders threaten to attack.

That learning happens through challenges. Skirmishes with the outside world educate the immune system and prompt it to build up its defenses. But that kind of cellular tough love means pushing our immune system beyond its comfort zone.

By oversanitizing our homes, the theory goes, and insulating our lives from natural dirt, we deny our immune system that chance. A disinfected environment means no exposure to germs, which in turn denies our immune sentries the chance to become stronger. If they don't encounter foreign microbes, blood cells that would normally differentiate between threatening invaders and innocent guests never have a chance to become trained at their job. As a result, our immune systems remain weak, unable to ward off infections and confused about when to attack and when to stand down. The use of bleach, antibacterial soap, and other cleansers in combination with children spending less time simply getting dirty may have contributed to increased rates of eczema, dry skin, multiple sclerosis, Crohn's disease, type 1 diabetes, asthma, hay fever, and, yes, allergies—so the theory goes.

Before we decide whether or not the hygiene hypothesis solves the food allergy mystery, some history may be useful. The idea originated with the British Cohort Study, an attempt to collect health information on all 16,567 British children born in one week in 1970. One analysis of the data uncovered an interesting phenomenon: The prevalence of eczema and hay fever was tied to the number of children in a family. The more siblings, the lower the incidence of both conditions.

British epidemiologist David Strachan took the next step. He counted up the occurrence of hay fever in 17,415 British children born during one week in 1958. According to his 1989 report, family size and birth order were more strongly linked to hay fever than any other factor. Children with older siblings were less likely to have hay fever at ages 11 and 23 than either only children or those who were the oldest brother or sister. Eczema was also tied to the number of older children in a home: more older siblings, less eczema. The phenomenon became known as the sibling effect. Strachan theorized that "unhygienic contact" between siblings might explain his observation: infections among the older children exposed the younger child and enabled her or him to build immunity to those germs.

Strachan offered this tentative explanation: "Over the past century declining family size, improvements in household amenities, and higher standards of personal cleanliness have reduced the opportunity for cross infection in young families. This may have resulted in more widespread clinical expression of atopic disease, emerging earlier in wealthier people." These words became distilled into what we now know as the hygiene hypothesis—our increased cleanliness is responsible for our diminished immune systems. The more infections the body experiences, the less likely we are to develop the immune disorders known as allergies.

In the years following these initial reports, numerous studies sought to document whether the sibling effect truly existed. Studies reported links between having older siblings and a lower incidence of asthma and even diabetes. Children who attend day care during the first six months of life may be at lower risk for asthma and eczema. In 2002, two epidemiologists at Michigan State University reviewed all of the data accrued to that point. All of the seventeen studies looking at hay fever incidence found the same inverse relationship: more siblings, less hay fever. Nine of the eleven studies on eczema reported the same phenomenon, as did twenty-one of the thirty-one studies looking at asthma and wheezing. The hypothesis grew to encompass not only hay fever and eczema but also many more immune conditions, including food allergy.

The idea was interesting, but no proof existed. If we became mildly infected with bacteria or viruses just by living in a less sanitary environment, and this mild infection left us immune to these microbes, then the immune system had to have some mechanism to make this happen. But science knew of no such mechanism.

So laboratory researchers began looking for one. Researchers in Italy suggested that some infections activate a type of immune cell called T helper 1, or Th1. Less exposure to germs means less Th1 activity, which in turn triggers other immune cells—T helper 2, or Th2—to awaken. And an abundance of Th2 activity is, it turns out, a feature of allergies.

Germany gave the hygiene hypothesis its next boost. In the 1980s, researchers found that children living in coal- and wood-heated homes in small villages in the Bavarian countryside had peculiarly low rates of allergies. That finding seems to contradict what we know about the serious health risks of these types of heating. Some epidemiologists figured that the rural air was still relatively cleaner air compared to urban areas like Munich and that this difference must be responsible for the lower allergy occurrence. But the research on that didn't bear out. All the data showed that children living on farms and with older siblings had lower rates of allergies, but no research pinpointed why.

Between 1999 and 2002, several studies pointed to a new possible target: a molecule found in bacteria called endotoxin. Research suggests that endotoxin flips an essential switch in the immune system known as TLR4. Importantly, the molecule is plentiful in the natural environment. In a study of more than 2,200 children in Austria, researchers looked at numerous factors to explain why children on farms were less likely to have hay fever or asthma compared with children raised elsewhere—living conditions, infections, diet, and pet exposure. The only variable that mattered was how often the children on farms had come into contact with livestock. As it turns out, endotoxin levels are high on farms. One study of 84 farming and non-farming households in Bavaria and Switzerland found that stables had the highest levels of endotoxin. That work also reported that the mattresses of the farm children had more endotoxin than the mattresses of nonfarm children. In 2001, the Allergy and Endotoxin (ALEX) Study, which studied 2,618 grade school children in rural Austria, Germany, and Switzerland, found that children who were around stables and drank farm milk during their first year of life were less likely to develop asthma and hay fever than children without these features in their earliest months.

To see if the story was the same indoors, researchers from Colorado got out their vacuum and collected dust from the living rooms, kitchens, and bedrooms of the homes of 61 babies who had been to the doctor for wheezing at least three times. Endotoxin levels were notably lower in the homes of infants with allergy issues compared to the homes of infants with no such issues. "Indoor endotoxin exposure early in life may protect against allergen sensitization," the researchers concluded. Endotoxin became the pillar holding up the hygiene hypothesis—where large amounts of this molecule swirled, allergies remained minimal.

The hygiene hypothesis may seem like a tidy explanation for the rise in food allergy and other immune disorders. And it may in fact be a contributing factor. But the evidence isn't conclusive, and many scientists disagree with this theory. Recent research contradicts it. Take the assertion that low Th1 activity leads to increased Th2 activity and thus allergy. Dutch researchers investigating allergies in

Gabon found high levels of Th2 without high rates of allergies. Other studies found that conditions thought to stem from a decrease in Th1—the cells that are supposed to protect us—are actually triggered by an increase instead. Also problematic is the finding that parasitic worms known as helminths trigger Th2 activity and yet thwart allergies, a further hitch in the theory. And respiratory viruses, such as rhinovirus and RSV (respiratory syncytial virus), don't protect against allergy and have instead been found to increase the risk of both allergies and asthma.

Contradicting evidence also surrounds the benefits of endotoxin and farm life. Some studies show that farm life is a risk factor for allergy and asthma. Other studies have simply failed to replicate the findings showing a protective effect. The same goes for endotoxin. Still other work shows that the link between endotoxin and allergy is filled with shades of gray: the timing of exposure, genetics, and the health of the individual, to name a few. Also, endotoxin can be harmful. Inhalation of the molecule can lead to chest tightness, fever, and inflammation. It can cause problems in the lungs and lead to asthma and wheezing that isn't tied to the immune system. About ten years after he suggested the link that snowballed into the hygiene hypothesis, David Strachan noted that the balance of evidence doesn't really support the idea that contacts outside the home in early childhood help prevent allergy.

In our estimation, the hygiene hypothesis isn't the complete solution to the mystery of food allergy. It's crucial to note that the studies behind the theory don't focus on food allergy. And although the nitty-gritty workings of the immune system may be the same for hay fever, eczema, and food allergy, the triggers may not be the same. Even if endotoxin helps prevent hay fever, that doesn't mean it helps prevent food allergy.

Still, we believe that the hygiene hypothesis holds some absolutely vital clues for understanding food allergy—and importantly, its prevention. And contemplating the hygiene hypothesis brings us to one of our core messages when it comes to understanding food allergy: the answer is rarely the same for everyone. Genetics, environment, upbringing, eating habits, and so much more contribute to the full picture of each individual with food allergy. Food allergy prevention and treatment isn't a one-size-fits-all practice. We'll delve into all this in upcoming chapters. But first let's look at other potential explanations for the food allergy epidemic.

OLD FRIENDS

Several years ago, British microbiologist Graham Rook proposed another hypothesis to explain the rise in immune disorders: old friends. The notion is similar to the hygiene hypothesis, but focuses on the gut microbiome, the collection of bacteria colonizing our digestive system.

Mounting research is revealing the importance of our gut microbiome to our overall health. This collection of "flora" influences our brains, our immune systems, and our ability to withstand numerous diseases. And it may play a role in food allergy.

The "old friends" theory begins with the fact that people living in the Western world aren't exposed to the same microbes that they have been throughout human evolution. We are constantly exposed to microbes that colonize our gut—in the womb, at the playground, at the dinner table, when we're sharing toys, when we're getting licked by the dog. These microorganisms also inhabit our skin and the environment we move through each day. They help educate the immune system, Rook theorized, bestowing it with a safe, balanced response to foreign substances. The parasitic worms that confound the hygiene hypothesis might be the exact kind of organism Rook was talking about. Fewer microbes make for an incomplete immune education. It's not the disease-causing microbes but rather the harmless ones that keep us protected from allergies.

Diversity matters. Research in the years since Rook first proposed his theory have opened our eyes to how important it is to expose ourselves to a wide array of microorganisms. That goes especially for infants. Many studies have found a tie between a diverse microbiome and our ability to withstand allergy disorders. In a study of 856 children, Anna Nowak-Wegrzyn, a pediatric allergist and immunologist at NYU Langone Hospital, and colleagues uncovered a powerful connection between a diverse diet and less asthma. Every additional food a child ate during the first year of life reduced the asthma risk by an additional 26 percent. Children with a less diverse diet had more food allergies by age 6, but most starkly by age 1.

Modern living, it seems, has compromised our dietary diversity. And here's where the hygiene hypothesis returns. Just as we've become less likely to suffer certain serious illnesses as a result of our more sanitary environment, we've also become less likely to encounter the same broad spectrum of bacteria that we once did.

But it's not just the sanitary environment of the twenty-first century that has reduced our exposure to a diverse array of microbes. It's our diet, which is not as high in diversity-protecting fiber as it once was. It's our use of antibiotics, which kill both the unhealthy bacteria making us sick and the healthy bacteria colonizing our gut. It's a lack of exposure to animals, which offer us their own host of microbes dwelling on their fur and their paws. It's a lot of things.

The outside world of microbes and the inside world of immunity are profoundly connected. A group led by University of Chicago food allergy researcher Cathy Nagler found that mice fed gut bacteria from human babies with allergies to milk developed the same allergy. Gut bacteria from infants who were healthy and without milk allergy protected mice against allergic reactions to milk. And a study by Talal Chatila at Boston Children's Hospital suggested that certain bacteria identified as beneficial to humans could protect mice from food allergy. In some of the animals, food allergy that was already present was reversed with the introduction of "good" bacteria.

The Broad Institute, a research center that is part of both Harvard and MIT, launched a years-long, multi-country study called DIABIMMUNE. Researchers are studying the gut flora of people in Russia, Finland, and Estonia, which offer distinct views on how the cultural environment may influence our gut microbiome. Although the northeastern Karelia region of Russia borders Finland, the two areas have starkly different economies. The geographic proximity and disparate lifestyles of these countries are ideal—a "living laboratory," as the researchers call it—for investigating how the way we live shapes our gut microbiomes and, in turn, our immune response. In other words, it may be a very effective way to study the hygiene hypothesis.

In recent years, some researchers have called for an end to the term *hygiene hypothesis*. The concern is well founded: poor hygiene has caused, and continues to cause, untold suffering. Many doctors fear that spreading the notion that hygiene is somehow bad for us will lead to a decrease in lifesaving practices such as handwashing. Let's be clear: Handwashing and other forms of hygiene are the best way to stop the spread of illness, period. Wash your hands. Have your children wash their hands. Relatives should wash their hands before holding your baby. So should your pediatrician. Stopping this practice isn't going to halt the incidence of type 1 diabetes, Crohn's disease, allergy, or any other immune disorder.

Hygiene per se isn't the problem, which makes the name misleading. Changes in how we live—away from animals, away from dirt, with an excessive use of antibiotics and a diet lacking a variety of plants—are the culprit behind our diminished microbiome. Birth by cesarean section may also curb microbiome diversity (more on this later). The formerly vibrant world of gut flora is now failing to steer our immune systems in the right direction. Food allergy is among the wrong turns our bodies are now taking more and more often.

But much remains to be understood still, and just like the hygiene hypothesis, the old friends theory isn't a complete answer. Genetics influences our susceptibility to allergic disorders, as well as our gut flora. And scientists still don't fully understand why diversity at the start of life is so important. As many readers will already be aware of, the health benefits of probiotics taken during childhood or adulthood are still undergoing research, although studies looking at their ability to thwart allergies are ongoing. Still, we stand by the notion that diversity, obtained through both diet and environmental exposure, is important for a healthy gut microbiome and is yet another crucial piece of the food allergy puzzle.

DUAL-ALLERGEN EXPOSURE THEORY

It may sound strange, but eating may not be the act that triggers food allergy at all. A growing body of evidence indicates that the skin may pose just as much of a risk, a finding that has led to the dual-allergen exposure theory.

This notion begins with the skin condition known as atopic dermatitis, or eczema. The red, itchy skin—common in children—arises from a cluster of factors, including immune function and the environment. Its role in food allergy stems from the fact that eczema makes the skin permeable. Normally our skin acts as a barrier, keeping out potentially harmful microbes and allergens. A protein known as FLG plays a crucial role in maintaining this barrier. But in people with eczema, FLG is often dysfunctional. As a result, the skin is not as strong a shield as it would otherwise be. When the skin is compromised in this way, proteins from foods left on tables or hands or even in dust can seep into the body. Immune system cells respond, triggering an allergic response. And when the individual then consumes the food by mouth, that response is at the ready.

The dual-allergen exposure theory explains the documented link between eczema and food allergy. Allergies come in many forms, including eczema, allergic asthma, hay fever (also called allergic rhinoconjunctivitis), and food allergy. Together, these constitute the "atopic" diseases, from the Greek word *atopy*, meaning "different." And they are all connected. Dry skin typically appears first, often arising during infancy or early childhood. Many infants with dry skin and/or eczema turn out to also have food allergies, and then hay fever and asthma often happen later, a progression referred to as the allergic march, or atopic march. This march varies considerably.

Some people outgrow their early allergies, and cases can be severe or mild—and there's no way to predict the course the march will take in a given individual. But research so far suggests that the march begins with eczema, and that the openings in the skin caused by this condition may be the first entry point for many food proteins that become allergens.

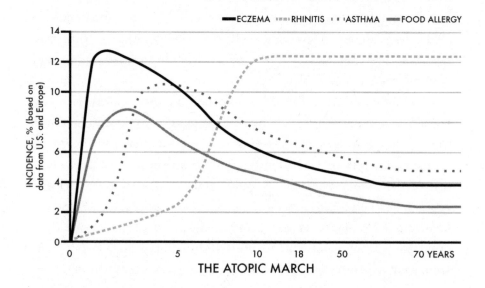

THE ATOPIC MARCH

Allergy researchers in the UK note that the dual-exposure hypothesis explains why rates of particular food allergies differ around the world: if a food isn't in the environment, then people with eczema aren't exposed to it through the skin. Where a food is common, environmental exposure will be, too. As we'll explain later, introducing foods early through the mouth can make all the difference.

Studies in animals have lent support to the dual-exposure theory. A study by researchers at Harvard and the University of Pennsylvania found skin lesions similar to eczema were tightly tied to food allergy in mice. The researchers also found that mice with injured skin had expanded and activated mast cells, a type of immune cell integral to food allergy reactions. In another investigation, researchers introduced peanut or ovalbumin (egg white protein) to rough skin patches on mice without functioning FLG. The mice developed severe responses to the foods. Other mouse studies have found the same reaction to egg white protein among mice with FLG mutations similar to those seen in people with eczema, whereas mice with normal FLG had no reaction.

Researchers have also seen the phenomenon in humans. Back in 1998, Dutch researchers found immune cells targeted against certain foods on the skin of a 6-month-old boy with eczema. In 2003, a UK team reported that children whose skin had been exposed to a little bit of peanut oil were at increased risk for peanut allergy by the time they were 5 years old. A group of French researchers found that 32 percent of children who had used skin cream containing oat had become allergic to this food. All of these studies supported the idea that the skin was somehow connected with food allergy.

The British team scrutinized exposure routes most carefully in a 2009 study that tracked how many peanuts mothers ate during pregnancy, breastfeeding, and their baby's first year of life. They also looked at the peanut-consuming habits among the rest of each child's household family members. The researchers found that in the homes of babies with peanut allergy, household members were eating far more peanuts than in the homes of babies without this allergy. They saw a direct connection between environmental exposure and peanut allergy: the greater the exposure, the higher the chance of allergy. It may even be that the concern about consuming common allergens during breastfeeding isn't so much about what the mother eats, but what proteins fall on the baby's skin as a result.

Lucky for baby, that's not an impossible problem to solve. We'll talk about how to do that later.

VITAMIN D

A deficiency in vitamin D appears to be yet another contributor to our risk of food allergy. We know that our skin produces vitamin D when it's exposed to the sun, leading some researchers to think that spending too much time indoors is responsible for increased rates of allergy and asthma. Simply living in a sunny place could also matter. In the United States and Australia, people living farthest from the equator bear the highest risk for food allergy. One study found that prescriptions for EpiPens to treat allergic reactions were higher in the northernmost states in the U.S. (less sun exposure) than in the southern states (more sun exposure); prescriptions in New England averaged 8 to 12 per 1,000 people, compared to 3 per 1,000 in southern regions of the country. Areas with more epinephrine prescriptions also have a lower incidence of melanoma, and vice versa, again hinting at some tie to sunlight exposure.

Birth season correlates with the likelihood of developing food allergy, another finding that boosts the vitamin D connection. A 2011 study from Australia found that the odds of a child developing food allergy was 55 percent lower for those born in summer compared to other seasons. A subsequent study confirmed that finding, noting that children born in autumn and winter had higher rates of food allergy and EpiPen prescriptions compared to children born in summer and spring.

We also have more direct data linking vitamin D deficiency to allergy risk. One Australian study found a stark difference between infants with low levels of vitamin D compared to those with sufficient levels: peanut allergy was eleven times more likely, egg allergy was four times more likely, and multiple allergy was at least ten times more likely in babies low in vitamin D. Other studies have hinted at a connection between vitamin D deficiency and food allergy, although the findings are often inconclusive. NHANES, which has tracked food allergy rates, says that peanut allergy is 2.39 times more likely among people low in vitamin D, but draws no such connection with egg or milk allergy. And there are data indicating that mothers who take vitamin D during pregnancy have babies with a lower risk of food reactions.

But the data are contradictory. Some studies have pointed to the opposite connection—that too much vitamin D is the problem. That insight originates with children raised on farms, where allergy is less common but where the use of vitamin supplements is, too. Supplemental vitamin D is often given to infants to prevent rickets, and throughout childhood to help bone growth. When researchers in Europe realized that farming communities there weren't using vitamin D supplements as aggressively as other places, they wondered if that difference contributed to the lower rates of allergic disorders among children raised on farms. Some research suggested that vitamin D may actually obstruct the natural Th1 immune response. A Finnish study found that by age 31, people who'd taken vitamin D supplements since infancy had higher rates of food allergy. In 2016, a group of German researchers reported that infants with the highest vitamin D levels at birth also had the highest food allergy rates by age 3. Another German group concluded that mothers with high vitamin D rates at birth had babies with a higher risk of food allergy, although other studies looking for the same connection haven't found it.

It may be a Goldilocks scenario: both too little vitamin D and too much vitamin D are problematic. Unpacking the cellular mechanisms behind these links is helping us understand what happens to our immune systems when we step out into the sunlight, spend long winters indoors, or drink milk fortified with vitamin D. Vitamin D may change the composition of our gut microbiome, and it appears to act on certain genes related to immunity. Based on the data thus far, we believe that the link between vitamin D deficiency and food allergy is strong enough to warrant consideration.

HOW FOOD ALLERGY WORKS

Having delved into the harrowing numbers and unraveled the possible explanations for the food allergy epidemic, it's time to understand how food allergy works. And that requires a trip to the microscopic world of the immune system.

As a reminder from chapter 1, we are focusing on reactions triggered by antibodies called immunoglobulin E, or IgE. Families coping with food allergy will often hear the term *IgE-mediated food allergy*.

These are the most common types of food allergies and the ones responsible for the reactions we typically associate with food allergy. Food sensitivities are not the same as food allergy (more on that below). Here we are speaking about a diagnosable, testable, and dangerous immune disease called food allergy.

The science behind food allergy can be daunting, but grasping the basics doesn't require a fancy degree or a deep knowledge of biology. The immune system is fascinating, complicated, and lifesaving. Understanding why it goes haywire in response to certain foods in some people may also leave us with a greater appreciation for all it does to keep us safe and healthy.

IgE antibodies were discovered in the mid-1960s by two different research groups simultaneously, one in Colorado and one in Sweden. In Colorado, husband and wife immunologists Kimishige and Teruko Ishizaka found an unidentified antibody through a series of experiments that began with the blood of a person with a severe allergy to ragweed pollen. In Sweden, immunochemists Hans Bennich and Gunnar Johansson homed in on the same antibody in the blood of a multiple myeloma patient. The two groups joined forces in 1968 to persuade the scientific powers that be to officially name their mystery antibody IgE. The discovery of IgE is a defining moment in the history of allergy research.

The Ishizakas continued to study IgE in the late 1960s and 1970s, now in their laboratory at Johns Hopkins University in Baltimore. They wanted to understand how the antibody leads to the release of histamine, a chemical that triggers the bodily reactions we typically associate with allergies—sneezing, itching, swelling. And they wanted to know exactly how the antibody worked inside the immune system. Meanwhile in Sweden, Johansson and his team were creating techniques to help researchers find ways to separate IgE from histamine as a way to treat allergy.

The thousands of studies spawned by these early findings have painted an intricate picture of how allergy works. Work by many research teams has brought this once-hidden world to light. When an allergen enters the body, IgE attaches to mast cells, which sit at the boundary between our tissues and the outside environment, as well as other types of cells. The next time the allergen appears (through a person eating the food it comes from), it encounters the mast cells with its specific IgE all over the body. That encounter coaxes the cells to release histamine; along with chemicals called cytokines, which cause inflammation; a variety of enzymes; and other compounds that contract muscles, including those governing our airways and force the body into other uncomfortable and unsafe states; all with the goal of pushing the dangerous food out of the body. The binding of IgE to mast cells and the activity that causes are at the heart of the allergic reaction that we see from the outside.

Researchers still don't know exactly why certain foods cause the immune system to produce IgE antibodies in the first place. We know that the body creates antibodies specific to each invader; every time we become infected with a new kind of bacteria, the body makes a unique antibody for that microbe. The next time that invader tries to gain entry, the immune system recognizes its antigens, compounds that stand like flagpoles on its surface, and prepares to fight to the death using antibodies. But these fights are typically waged with IgG antibodies, which exist in much greater number than IgE antibodies. IgE antibodies to allergens are different. They are often involved in the atopic march—eczema (or atopic dermatitis), "hay fever" (or allergic rhinitis), allergic asthma. But science hasn't gotten to the bottom of why a harmless food would be misread as an enemy in the first place.

Studies have generated some ideas. We know that it's the protein in an allergen that causes the problem. Among the threats that are ingested, the proteins often share certain traits—they're small, their structure is unchanged by cooking, they easily separate from the rest of the allergen, and they do their bidding in very low doses. Researchers have shown that just a tiny amount of an allergen landing on mucosal tissue (like the inside of the mouth) is enough to launch an IgE response. Enzymes, a type of protein, seem especially

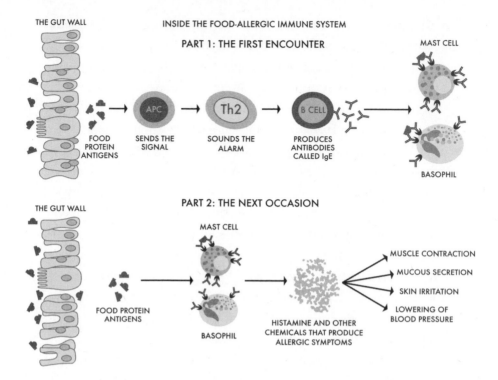

INSIDE THE FOOD-ALLERGIC IMMUNE SYSTEM

PART 1: THE FIRST ENCOUNTER

THE GUT WALL

MAST CELL

FOOD PROTEIN ANTIGENS → SENDS THE SIGNAL (APC) → SOUNDS THE ALARM (Th2) → PRODUCES ANTIBODIES CALLED IgE (B CELL)

BASOPHIL

PART 2: THE NEXT OCCASION

THE GUT WALL

MAST CELL

FOOD PROTEIN ANTIGENS

BASOPHIL

HISTAMINE AND OTHER CHEMICALS THAT PRODUCE ALLERGIC SYMPTOMS

MUSCLE CONTRACTION
MUCOUS SECRETION
SKIN IRRITATION
LOWERING OF BLOOD PRESSURE

Normally when the body encounters a new type of food protein, the immune system learns to recognize and tolerate it without problem. Food allergy follows a different chain of events. In this scenario, when food protein antigens, or markers, pass through the gut wall for the first time (Part 1), antigen-presenting cells (APC) send a signal to an immune cell called a type 2 T helper cell (Th2). A Th2 cell in turn alerts the B cells, which start the production of IgE antibodies (Y-shaped structures). These IgE antibodies attach to mast cells and basophils. The next time that food protein antigen shows up, the IgE antibodies attached to mast cells and basophils spring into action, producing histamine and other chemicals that produce the reactions we know as allergy symptoms.

adept at provoking Th2, the immune cell involved in many allergic reactions, which in turn calls IgE into action. Papain, an enzyme in papaya that is used as a meat tenderizer, is known to trigger an allergic reaction in people who prepare it, for example.

Genetics may also factor in. A wide range of environmental allergens cause IgE responses in up to 40 percent of Western populations. This group of people tends to have higher amounts of IgE circulating in their blood than other people. Research suggests that several genes could be involved in determining who will be part of that 40 percent. Studies have uncovered a few possible genes that may be food allergy risk factors, and the evidence that genetics plus the surrounding environment (a combination known as epigenetics) influences the likelihood of food allergy is persuasive. But the research is still inconclusive, and when it comes to genetics, the picture is almost always complex. Environment matters. Timings matter. Other genes matter.

Whatever it is that sets off the immune system to produce IgE, we know what happens next. The antibody sticks to mast and other cells and causes an allergic reaction. When the allergen in a food meets its IgE antibody attached to mast cells, the antibody makes the mast cells release chemicals that can lead to mild reactions like hives, moderate reactions like stomachache, or severe reactions like wheezing. Ultimately the body may enter anaphylaxis, a state of shock in which the airways narrow, the blood pressure drops, and the pulse weakens. The person may vomit and will soon have trouble breathing unless they get a shot of epinephrine, which halts the process. In some cases, the story ends tragically, as it did with Natalie Giorgi. Most times, the allergic episode ends with recovery. But even a mild allergic reaction can be traumatizing, leaving people fearful of their next restaurant outing, their next undisclosed ingredient on a packaged food, their next brush with a contaminated lunch tray. And a minor reaction one day doesn't guarantee a minor reaction in the future.

Despite the many questions still remaining about food allergy, we know for sure that once the body is geared to react to a food, it's difficult to convince it otherwise. Our research group at Stanford and many other researchers around the globe have spent the last two decades developing safe and effective methods to teach the body a new trick: seeing these proteins not as allergens but as foods. At the very least, these approaches are making formerly hazardous foods safe to eat in small amounts, so that if an allergic person does accidentally consume a bit, the threat of harm is erased. The programs for ending the food allergy epidemic, presented in upcoming chapters, are changing lives in both big and subtle ways. At the same time, scientists have parsed the mechanisms driving allergic reactions down to their many working parts, providing an ever-expanding number of opportunities for creating drugs that could throw a wrench in the allergy clockwork. All of this work has created the dawn of a new era for those who've been diagnosed with food allergy.

OTHER ALLERGIC-TYPE REACTIONS

Eosinophilic esophagitis: Along with food allergy, a condition known as eosinophilic esophagitis, or EoE, is also on the rise, though less dramatically. With EoE, immune cells called eosinophils are found in the esophagus, where they are not normally located. In severe cases, this extra material can cause the esophagus to narrow to the point where food becomes stuck, requiring immediate medical attention. Research suggests that EoE is associated with food allergy, but the nature of that link is not well understood, especially because EoE cannot be detected by measuring IgE levels. It is unknown if immunotherapy to treat food allergy can induce permanent EoE, or if certain types of immunotherapy may be part of the solution for someone with both food allergy and EoE.

Food protein–induced enterocolitis syndrome: A condition known as food protein–induced enterocolitis syndrome, or FPIES, is another type of allergy. As the name suggests, FPIES is tied to food, but its inner workings differ from food allergy and it can't be diagnosed using food allergy tests. The condition usually occurs in infants and toddlers and can cause vomiting, diarrhea, and dehydration, all of which can become severe, but it often resolves on its own by the time a child is 5 years of age. Milk, soy, rice, oat, and egg are the most common triggers. No specific tests for FPIES exist and thus we don't know much about its prevalence.

Oral allergy syndrome: Pollen also has a strange connection to food allergy. In a syndrome known as oral allergy syndrome, the proteins that trigger a reaction to pollen also trigger a reaction to certain raw fruits and vegetables. Individuals with hay fever caused by a protein in birch may be allergic to apple. Latex allergy may occur alongside allergy to kiwi, tomato, or bell pepper. The symptoms caused by oral allergy syndrome are usually the worst during pollen season and typically occur only with the raw food, not food that's been cooked, because heat alters the protein.

Alpha gal allergy: Allergies to meat have always been uncommon—until recently. A strange syndrome tied to a carbohydrate (called galactose-alpha-1,3-galactose) appears to trigger meat allergy following bites by certain species of ticks. With this allergy, known as alpha gal and identified by Thomas Platts-Mills at the University of Virginia, people bitten by a tick may suffer mild to severe allergy symptoms several hours after eating red meat. Many researchers are trying to figure out the mechanism behind this allergy.

MORE ABOUT INTOLERANCE AS OPPOSED TO ALLERGIES

We've already distinguished between food intolerance and food allergies. But because adverse reactions to certain foods have drawn increasing attention, it's worth digging into this topic a bit deeper. Recent years have seen a spike in concern about certain foods. Gluten—the mix of proteins that makes bread dough stretchy and is found in wheat, rye, barley, and other grains—bears the brunt of this concern. The burgeoning market of gluten-free foods, bakeries, and restaurant offerings is impossible to miss. The market for these products in the United States exceeds $6.5 billion annually. Dairy is another common source of complaint. Some people can't eat peppers; others can't tolerate strong spices. Food additives are sometimes the culprit.

Just because these adverse reactions are hard to diagnose medically does not mean the reactions are imaginary. Each of us consumes about 100 tons of food in a lifetime. That's 100 tons for a gastrointestinal tract to process. Clearly, the digestive system is expertly honed to handle the range of proteins, sugars, and fats we send its way throughout our lives. The body's general compliance with our diet means that when digestion doesn't go smoothly, we should listen.

The inability to tolerate one food or another is far more common than food allergy. Up to 20 percent of Americans experience discomfort after eating their food nemesis. But these reactions are rarely severe or dangerous. Food intolerance is not an immune disorder. There is no wrangling of IgE, no calling in the troops of mast cells, no firing of chemical weapons at the enemy. Rather, food intolerance typically appears as bloating, gas, and other gastrointestinal discomfort. These reactions aren't pleasant, but they are usually short-lived and confined to the digestive system.

The causes of food intolerance differ from those of food allergy. A gastrointestinal tract can become damaged. Infections may interrupt digestion. Sometimes digestive issues sound the alarm for more serious underlying conditions such as inflammatory bowel disease or Crohn's disease. The body may be having a difficult time absorbing carbohydrates. Medication may be interfering with the body's ability to digest a certain food. And much of the world is unable to digest lactose, a sugar in milk.

Tests for food intolerance differ from those for food allergy. A doctor may take a stool sample or a urine sample or do a breath test to trace a particular discomfort back to a food. Some tests are more involved, and all are crucial for ruling out serious diseases. Tests are now available that can discern between food intolerance, food allergy, and celiac disease. However, it's still crucial to consult an allergy specialist when pursuing any testing for these issues. Some diagnostics can be faulty and also may not be covered by insurance, which means wasted out-of-pocket spending. As for treatment, some intolerance can be managed simply by avoiding the food. Other times they warrant medical attention. Some bad reactions result from eating disorders, which require serious and immediate attention from a health professional.

These days it can sometimes seem that everyone has some food issue. It can even seem to be a trend rather than an actual phenomenon. For those suffering from genuine IgE-mediated food allergy, complaints of gluten sensitivity can seem to draw attention away from more serious life-threatening health issues. But the rise in food-related complaints has likely been a benefit to those coping with food allergy. Restaurants are far more likely to consider allergies than they were a decade ago. Food allergy is no longer treated like a fake disease. And both allergy and intolerance draw attention to issues with our modern food supply—our reliance on processed food, our overuse of antibiotics, and potential health risks associated with pesticides. Food allergy sufferers should learn to see their food-intolerance pals as allies in the quest for safer and healthier diets.

THE BOTTOM LINE

- Food allergy rates have increased globally over the past few decades and continue to do so. Up to 8 percent of children and 11 percent of adults worldwide have food allergy.

- No single theory explains this trend. Scientists currently believe a combination of factors is responsible. Modern living curbs the ability of our immune system to distinguish between harmful and harmless substances. And initial exposure to food allergens through the skin may lead to food allergy.

- Antibodies known as IgE are behind the reactions we know of as food allergy. However, it is possible to have elevated IgE levels without actually being allergic, a phenomenon known as food sensitivity.

- A person may be unable to tolerate a food without being allergic. Food intolerance is a real condition, though usually less severe than food allergy.

Chapter 3

IS IT MY FAULT? ESCAPING THE BLAME GAME

Replacing guilt with evidence-based insights about food allergy risk factors

Brynna Gianos wasn't new to parenting. But her experience wasn't enough to quell her nerves as she stood in our San Francisco pediatric allergy clinic one Friday morning, holding her 6-month-old daughter, Auden, on the examination table. Auden had developed a rash around her mouth after her first taste of eggs, and Brynna, worried that the reaction would be more severe next time, wanted her daughter tested. A knot of worry strained her otherwise cheerful demeanor. "I ate an omelet pretty much every day of my pregnancy," she said. "And I had a C-section." Now she blamed herself for a food allergy that could transform her daughter's life before it even gets started. She was trying to play it cool, but her guilt seeped through. Brynna sounded like so many other parents of children with food allergy: all too ready to accuse and criticize themselves for no reason.

New parents rarely escape the concern that their newborn may have a food allergy. Horror stories and warnings are too ubiquitous these days to feed our children dairy or peanuts with our caution thrown freely to the wind. Given the rising rates of food allergy, the concern is warranted. Less justified, though, is the guilt that many parents suffer when a child tests positive. Did they inherit it from me? What should I have done differently? How could I have stopped this? Why did I have to crave eggs so much?

It's impossible to say why the skin around Auden's mouth turned blotchy after that first taste. But it wasn't Brynna's penchant for omelets while her daughter was in the womb. For all that we *don't* know about food allergy, we have enough evidence to assuage the blame. And we have enough information to help parents make sensible changes where and when it's possible and to exercise appropriate caution as their infants move from breast milk or formula to solid foods.

In this chapter, we will explore what we know about genes and food allergy, how the nine months of gestation may or may not heighten the risk of allergies, and what research has been done about the connection between cesarean sections and food allergy. And we'll outline the first steps to take if you fear you or your child may have a food allergy. The goal here is to exchange blame and guilt for common sense and empowering knowledge.

DO GENES MATTER?

The answer to this first and most obvious question is yes and no. Studies over the past two decades have illuminated the hidden ways in which our DNA may make us more prone to food allergy. But the findings aren't conclusive. There's no such thing as a "food allergy gene," and as to those genes that do seem to influence the risk, we aren't sure how or when they come into play. Several rare congenital syndromes give rise to food allergy, but these are the exceptional causes, not the rule. Still, knowing whether a food-allergic parent is more or less likely to have a food-allergic child—and knowing what genetic entanglements are completely random—may help families prepare and cope with a diagnosis.

Many studies have tackled the question of inheritance. Data from the HealthNuts study, a large investigation that included more than 5,000 infants in Australia, found that 10 percent of children with food allergy had no family history of the condition. That estimate may be low. In a 2016 study from Chicago that included 832 food-allergic children, 46 percent (291 children) had a mother and/or father with food allergy.

In an early attempt to figure out whether peanut allergy was inherited, research led by Scott Sicherer at the Icahn School of Medicine at Mount Sinai in New York recruited 58 pairs of twins among whom at least one member had a confirmed peanut allergy. Because some of the pairs shared all their genes (identical twins), some shared just half (fraternal twins), and the environment was the same for each pair, the researchers could calculate the hand that DNA had in the allergy. To do this, they used a statistic known as the concordance rate, which calculates the likelihood of both members of a twin pair having the same trait. By comparing the concordance rate of the identical twins to that of the fraternal twins, the researchers could figure out the likelihood that peanut allergy was inherited. This method had already been used to investigate the heritability of many diseases, including asthma and eczema, which are closely tied to food allergy. The study estimated that peanut allergy was about 82 percent inheritable. The genetic influence, the researchers concluded, was "significant." More recently, a group of Swedish researchers looked at data on asthma, eczema, and food allergy from more than 25,000 Swedish twins at age 9 or 12 years. "Asthma and allergic diseases of childhood are highly heritable," the 2016 paper stated.

Another way to find out whether food allergy is inherited is to look at entire families. Does having a parent or sibling with food allergy make it likelier that you will, too? The HealthNuts study looked at just that. Among more than 5,200 infants, those with one immediate family member who had food allergy were just a bit more likely to have the same condition than infants without that tie. But if two or more family members had food allergy, the infant's risk spiked. The researchers also uncovered some unexpected connections. Mothers who had battled asthma or eczema in their lives and siblings who'd had hay fever were each linked to egg allergy in the infant. Mothers and fathers with a history of asthma and hay fever were more likely to have infants with peanut allergy.

In the early 1990s, researchers on the Isle of Wight looked at all 1,456 children born on the island between January 1989 and February 1990 for peanut allergy, checking for the condition when the children were 1 year old, 2 years old, and 4 years old. They concluded that a family history of eczema and egg allergy influenced a child's likelihood of having peanut allergy. A group in Chicago looked at 581 nuclear families to see whether having a brother or sister with food allergy predicted whether a child would have the condition, too. And it did. According to the study, published in 2009, food allergy in one child was an independent risk factor—meaning no other variable mattered—for food allergy in another child in the family. Having a mother or father with food allergy was also strongly tied to the likelihood of food allergy in a child (though not as strong as the sibling link), and that held for peanut, wheat, milk, egg whites, soy, walnuts, shrimp, codfish, and sesame.

Our genes rarely act alone. They have help from the environment. The complex interplay between our genes and our surroundings varies for every condition. We know that certain chemicals in the environment can increase cancer risk by triggering certain genes to mutate, for example. But we don't know how much of that chemical it takes or who is most at risk for that particular trigger. Food allergy may work similarly. A second study of twins, this time of 826 pairs in rural China, concluded that both genes and the environment influence food allergy. Heritability was highest for people with peanut and shellfish allergies. Nongenetic factors that may have influenced food allergy include exposure to cigarette smoke, allergens like grass or pollen, and the individual's history of respiratory infections. Interestingly, in the HealthNuts study, parents born in East Asia had lower rates of food allergy compared to others in the study, yet had children with relatively higher rates of food allergy, pointing to an environmental factor.

Yet another study introduces some subtler considerations. Sometimes a child may test positive for food allergy but not actually react when they eat the food. The expansive Chicago Family Cohort Food Allergy study found that among the 1,120 children with food-allergic siblings, about half tested positive for food allergy but didn't have a reaction when they tried the actual food. And less than 14 percent of the children in this group had an allergic reaction to the food in question. That rate isn't much higher than the rate in the general population. Children with food-allergic siblings may test positive for the allergy but never react to the food. This insight offers parents a slower journey to the land of food allergy worries. A positive test doesn't always mean danger is lurking.

The heritability of food allergy is still being studied. We know that peanut allergy can be passed down from grandparent or parent to child, but we also know that this doesn't always happen. We know that food allergy may cluster within families, but we also know that just because one sibling has this disease, that doesn't mean the others will. However, the presence of food allergy within a nuclear family gives parents a reasonable starting point for caution.

When it comes to finding the specific genes responsible for inherited food allergy, studies of peanut allergy have led the way—and found villains buried in our DNA. Mutations in a gene called filaggrin that lead it to lose some of its function can result in peanut allergy, possibly by causing defects in our skin barrier. Changes in a group of genes known as the human leukocyte antigen (HLA) system, which encodes proteins that keep the immune system on track, are also related to peanut allergy. Another study of nearly 2,800 parents and children in the United States also found culprit sites in the HLA system.

A 2017 study pushed beyond peanuts. Geneticists in Germany and the United States examined the genomes of 1,500 children in both countries. Each of our 20,000 or so genes is made of a string of chemicals called nucleotides, signified as A, T, G, and C. Every time our cells divide, our DNA replicates—one copy for each cell. And during that replication, a change may happen to a letter in that string. These changes, known as single nucleotide polymorphisms, or SNPs, may become permanent. Sometimes they're harmless. Sometimes they aren't.

In the 2017 study, the researchers looked at more than 5 million SNPs. They discovered five specific locations on the human genome that are risk factors for food allergy. That is, certain changes at these five points increase a person's chance of developing food allergy. One of the regions involves genes related to the skin and the mucous membrane of the esophagus. And four of the five regions appeared to be tied to all food allergy, not just one or two specific foods.

Zeroing in on which neighborhoods in our genome are housing food allergy mutations may not be of much practical use yet. But finding these genes gives drug developers new targets and may also lead to new diagnostic tests. In time, they may also help explain the epidemic.

SOME GENES ASSOCIATED WITH FOOD ALLERGY

The following list is a selection of some genes that may be related to the cause of food allergy. Genes play a role in this condition sometimes. The interaction between genes and the surrounding environment (epigenetics) is likely more important when it comes to food allergy.

GENE	WHAT WE KNOW
HLA	Studies have linked various versions of this gene to peanut allergy.
Filaggrin	Mutated forms of this gene that lose their function may increase the risk of food allergy.
STAT6	A version of this gene has been linked to nut allergy.
IL-10	Milk allergy that does not resolve on its own has been tied to some forms of this gene.

IL-13	Just a single change in the code for this gene may trigger the immune system to become sensitized against certain food proteins.
SPINK5	Children with eczema may be more likely to develop food allergies with certain forms of this gene.
FOXP3	A change in this gene leads to severe food allergy related to a rare disease known as IPEX syndrome. This gene is also linked to immune-related asthma.
STAT3	After an anaphylaxis patient with this genetic mutation was found to have high levels of IgE, researchers wondered how this gene might be related to food allergy.*

*Muraro A, et al. Precision medicine in allergic disease-food allergy, drug allergy, and anaphylaxis-PRACTALL document of the European Academy of Allergy and Clinical Immunology and the American Academy of Allergy, Asthma, and Immunology. *Allergy*. 2017 Jul;72(7):1006–21.

THE FIRST ENVIRONMENT

The mixing and mingling of parental DNA may explain some newborn food allergy. But there may be other routes—namely, via the umbilical cord. Many new mothers begin worrying about the health of their babies from the moment the pregnancy test comes out positive. Out goes the caffeine, in come heaps of leafy greens. And as food allergy has become more common, so has the tendency to eliminate certain foods from pregnancy diets. Paranoia and too much Googling could lead many mothers to wonder if their nine-month cheese habit led to their baby's milk allergy.

The recent history surrounding the link between pregnancy diet and infant food allergies is entangled with the history of food allergy research as a whole. As our understanding of this disease has evolved, so has our thinking about what mothers should or shouldn't consume. We'll delve into that history in a later chapter because it provides essential context for the new era of preventing and treating food allergy. But for parents suffering from guilt, or pregnant women panicking in the supermarket, the facts offer a sigh of relief.

In 2000, the American Academy of Pediatrics recommended that pregnant women avoid peanuts as a way to reduce the risk of peanut allergy in the growing fetus. That recommendation came in the form of a single sentence at the end of a publication focused on infant formula and breastfeeding. "No maternal dietary restrictions during pregnancy are necessary," the Academy stated, "with the possible exception of excluding peanuts." But that was enough to send many expectant women fleeing from the peanut butter aisle. The notion that infants could develop food allergy based on what mothers ate while pregnant seeped into our collective consciousness, giving women one more worry, one more cause for guilt, one more reason to think they weren't doing it right.

Hints that maternal diet may not be the allergy driver many women came to fear already existed. In the 1980s, two Swedish researchers looked for atopy among infants whose mothers had avoided milk and eggs during pregnancy. Starting at halfway through their pregnancies, 212 women were randomized to either eat or abstain from these foods. After their babies were born, many of the newly breastfeeding mothers assigned to the allergen-free diet decided to keep their intake of milk and eggs low. But it turned out that allergies—eczema, asthma, hay fever, and food reactions—were equally common in both groups. Maternal diet, it seems, had little impact on the risk of food allergies.

Another Swedish study of 165 pregnant women with asthma as well as an allergy to pollen or animal dander tested different diets. The researchers randomly assigned the participants to one of four diets, ranging from no eggs or milk to one egg and a liter of milk per day during the last trimester. If maternal diet mattered, the researchers theorized, then the infants whose mothers ate eggs and drank milk should already have IgE antibodies to those foods at birth. But when they looked at the levels of IgE antibodies in the cord blood following birth, they found no differences.

Five years later, the researchers revisited the first study. Perhaps the difference between the two diet groups would take time to emerge, as babies grew into allergic toddlers. But among the 198 children they evaluated, those from the elimination arm of the study did not have fewer allergies. In fact, children from that group were actually more likely to be allergic to egg.

Not all the data exonerate peanuts during pregnancy. In 1999, a small study from South Africa found that expectant mothers who ate peanuts more than once a week raised the risk of peanut allergy for their newborn compared to those who ate peanuts less often. Another study, from the UK, looked for correlations between childhood food allergy and a host of family-related factors in 622 surveys. Eating peanuts during pregnancy appeared to increase the likelihood of peanut allergy in children less than 5 years of age, but not those older than 5 years. Both of these studies, however, were based on questionnaires that required mothers to recall how often they ate peanuts while they were pregnant, sometimes up to years later. That doesn't invalidate the studies, but it does raise caution about how wide to open our arms when we embrace the findings.

A shift began at the start of the twenty-first century when a group of British researchers turned to a massive bank of data for some better intelligence. The Avon Longitudinal Study of Parents and Children included almost 14,000 people, and allergists George du Toit, Gideon Lack, and colleagues plundered it for information on food allergy risk factors. Their 2003 study, published in *The New England Journal of Medicine*, found no link to prenatal diet among children with peanut allergy. As with earlier studies, this one was retrospective—mothers were answering questions about their prenatal diet long after the fact—which makes the results less robust than a randomized, prospective study.

In 2008, the American Academy of Pediatrics reversed course. Studies, the Academy pronounced, "have not supported a protective effect of a maternal exclusion diet." Abstaining from egg and milk during pregnancy would not help prevent food allergy in infants. And while acknowledging work showing that avoiding peanuts could help thwart the allergy in children, the Academy also pointed toward studies showing the opposite. The publication offered a clear summary: there's no persuasive evidence in favor of eliminating potential allergens from the prenatal diet.

A 2010 study came to the opposite conclusion. Among 140 infants with IgE antibodies to peanut, having a mother who ate peanuts while she was pregnant was a risk factor. As with some earlier studies, this one was based on a questionnaire that asked mothers to recall how much peanut they consumed during each trimester of their pregnancy—less than twice a week, twice a week or more but less than daily, daily, or unknown. The average age of the infants enrolled in the study was 9 months, which means some mothers were recalling how often they ate peanuts up to a year and a half earlier. As we've suggested, although one's pregnancy diet often becomes a nostalgic memory, that memory isn't always accurate. Also, the peanut allergy test used in this study indicated that the infants were sensitive, not that they reacted to the food; as noted earlier, the former doesn't always mean the latter. Still, the data in this study shouldn't be fully dismissed.

However, a comprehensive and rigorous Cochrane Review, an evidence-based overview by a UK-based nonprofit, inspected data from five trials with a total of 952 participants. That review focused mainly on the occurrence of asthma and eczema in children (both of which can be linked to the subsequent development of food allergy). The authors of that review called the evidence on whether a prenatal diet eschewing milk, eggs, or other potential allergens prevented asthma and eczema "inadequate."

All this research on the link between pregnancy diets and food allergy shows one fact very clearly: science isn't always clear-cut.

More often than not, the results are subtle or contradictory. It can be difficult for even the most seasoned expert to tease out the truth. We offer all this research not to confuse you but rather to equip you with the information.

At our center at Stanford University, we recommend that pregnant women and breastfeeding mothers maintain a nutritious diet made up of what they would like to eat. Diversifying the diet is key, as is not avoiding foods except those that are unhealthy (soda, candy, chips, and the like). The World Health Organization (WHO) recommends exclusive breastfeeding for the first few months of life, and that's a good guideline to follow. We also recommend nursing for as long as possible, if nursing is an option. In short, there's no need to shape your diet during pregnancy or breastfeeding around the fear of food allergies.

LIQUID LUNCH

This brings us to one of the first worries parents have once babies leave the womb: breastfeeding. We know that the nutrients from our diets seep into breast milk and thereby into our infants. So it's logical for a new mother to wonder whether the newly developed food allergy in her toddler derived from the peanuts she fueled herself with on the go, the eggs she inhaled for breakfast, or some other component of her diet.

Wading through the recommendations surrounding breastfeeding can be complicated and frustrating. They often mix evidence on what diet to follow while nursing with evidence on how long to nurse for, for example, leaving tired mothers at a loss for clear advice. And for mothers who give their infants formula instead of breast milk, reading the current research can feel like swimming through an ocean of finger-wagging waves. We suggest that new mothers consult with their pediatrician along with an allergist if there's a family history of food allergy and follow whatever course is best for them. Studies have found that nursing reduces the risk for food allergy compared to formula. According to the American Academy of Pediatrics, breastfeeding for at least four months reduces the risk of eczema and milk allergy for the first two years of life. Worldwide, health authorities recommend breastfeeding, partly to correct an unnecessary shift toward formula pushed by manufacturers in prior decades. But ultimately the decision of whether to nurse or use formula is personal.

With regard to whether the diet a nursing mother consumes has any bearing on her child's likelihood of food allergy, the trajectory of the research has been much the same as for the prenatal months. After earlier suggestions to avoid risky foods while lactating, medical authorities changed their views. Avoiding some food allergens may help prevent eczema in children, and some data point toward avoiding peanuts when babies are at high risk because the allergy is in the nuclear family. But taken as a whole, the data don't show that the mother's diet matters much in the quest to prevent food allergy. According to the same Cochrane Review that tackled prenatal diet, two studies with a total of 523 participants showed this lack of connection. At ages 1, 2, and 7 years old, children had the same incidence of milk, egg, and peanut allergy whether or not their mothers consumed those foods while pregnant. The reviewers called for larger and better clinical trials to tackle this question.

The international consensus on preventing food allergy by avoiding foods during pregnancy or nursing is clear: the evidence doesn't support that approach. In 2019, the American Academy of Pediatrics published an updated version of its recommendations on breastfeeding and allergy that advised against such dietary changes. The European Academy of Allergy and Clinical Immunology (EAACI) holds the same position. So does the Australasian Society of Clinical Immunology and Allergy (ASCIA).

WHAT ABOUT FORMULA?

Parents who choose to feed their newborns formula may feel stigmatized in light of the current recommendations to breastfeed exclusively for at least four months. However, when it comes to food allergy, the evidence that formula feeding increases the risk is unpersuasive. For parents feeding their newborns with formula, the most recent recommendation from both the AAP and EAACI is that using partially versus extensively hydrolyzed formula makes no difference when it comes to food allergy risk.

A 2008 study from Australia found that soy-based formula did not raise the risk of peanut intolerance, as earlier studies had suggested it did. Another large Australian study, this one from 2016, found no link between the duration of exclusive breastfeeding and the risk of food allergy at one year of age. This study also found no proof that partially hydrolyzed formula was better than milk formula at preventing food allergy.

As with so many areas of food allergy research, some studies reached an opposing conclusion. When researchers at the University of Memphis surveyed new mothers about how they fed their children during the first twelve months, they found a connection. Children who'd been given a combination of direct breast milk, pumped breast milk, and formula were more likely to develop food allergy symptoms during their first six years of life than children who'd been exclusively breastfed.

Taken as a whole, though, the evidence against formula is scarce. And there is no proof that so-called hypoallergenic formulas prevent food allergy. Parents giving their infants formula should consult their pediatricians or allergists if there is a family history of food allergy and if they are concerned about what product to use, or any other issue surrounding feeding during the first few months of life.

At our center, we recommend following the guidelines set by U.S. and European pediatric authorities, which advise that hypoallergenic formula is not helpful for preventing food allergy. We suggest breastfeeding as much as possible, supplementing with formula only if necessary—recognizing that sometimes it is. For those who are feeding their babies with formula, we suggest consulting with a pediatrician about which type offers the best vitamins and proteins for your infant.

THE EFFECT OF CESAREAN SECTION

Like Brynna, many parents of food-allergic children wonder whether C-sections increase the risk of food allergies. The answer is far from clear. The number of babies born by cesarean section around the world nearly doubled between 2000 and 2015. A survey of 169 countries published by *The Lancet* in 2018 found that 15 percent of all births were by cesarean in 106 of the surveyed countries, with a large portion being medically unnecessary. Putting reasons for choosing birth by cesarean aside, parents hoping to avoid food allergy in their children may want to consider the evidence surrounding the link between the two.

There is no cause for blame or shame here. Cesarean sections save lives. Mothers of children who were born by this method and who have food allergy do not need to feel guilty. As we will see, the evidence is not conclusive. And in the studies that have shown this link, the data are not that stark. Still, a body of research has emerged over the past decade indicating that the risk of food allergy could be increased by cesarean section birth. Some expecting parents may find it useful to include these findings in their considerations. And the research also touches some of the central questions surrounding food allergy—namely, how microbes, including beneficial bacteria, may protect against the condition.

A plethora of studies has probed the role of C-sections in food allergy. After identifying nearly 9,000 children with hay fever, asthma, eczema, or food allergy in a health records database, a group of researchers from Oregon matched up these diagnoses with birth records that included the type of delivery. Hay fever and asthma were more common in babies born by C-section, although the link in asthma was seen only with girls. But food allergy was a minor issue, affecting just 29 children in the study, less than half a percent of the cohort.

In 2008, researchers from Ireland investigated the link between childhood asthma, a risk factor for food allergy, and C-sections. They conducted a meta-analysis, a study of studies, typically considered the most rigorous type of investigation. According to their analysis of twenty-three prior reports, children delivered by C-section had a 20 percent increased risk of asthma.

Another meta-analysis homed in on food allergy along with several other allergic conditions. In their review of twenty-six studies conducted between 1966 and 2007, Danish researchers found that pinpointing the link between C-sections and food allergy is not simple. Many of the studies parsing this link were based on small numbers of children, and thus don't necessarily reflect the population as a whole. And many were plagued by large standard errors, a statistical figure that indicates the accuracy of a calculation. Standard error is akin to saying *give or take*—the larger the give or take, the less rigorous the data. Taken together, the small study size and the large standard error result in data that skew toward showing a stronger connection than may really exist. In this meta-analysis, the researchers concluded that this bias could easily explain the heightened risk of food allergy posed by cesarean births seen in prior studies.

But another analysis looking specifically at food allergy only did find an increased incidence among children born by C-section. In this meta-analysis, researchers from Australia focused on four studies in which food allergy had been diagnosed by either symptoms after eating the food or the presence of IgE antibodies targeting known food allergens in blood samples. In two studies that followed children from birth, babies born by C-section had IgE antibodies indicating food sensitivities more often than babies born by vaginal delivery. In two studies looking at food allergy diagnosed through an oral food challenge, one found no difference in prevalence between cesarean and vaginal delivery. But in the other study, parents reported food allergies by 2 years of age more often for children born by C-section. Importantly, this effect existed only for children born to mothers who themselves had food allergy. The researchers concluded that the link between cesarean births and food allergy was frail at best.

Another noteworthy study followed 512 children from birth through 2 years of age to see if delivery route made any difference in the likelihood of food allergy. Of the 512 births, 171 were by C-section and 341 were vaginal. By age 2, 35 children had been diagnosed with some kind of food reaction, though just 8 had an IgE-mediated allergy. And according to the results, the food allergy group did not include a disproportionately large fraction of C-section deliveries.

Understanding why cesarean delivery could increase the risk of food allergy means returning to the gut microbiome. In the 1990s, allergy researchers around the world noticed something peculiar: Central and Eastern Europe had lower rates of atopic diseases than Western Europe. No one knew why, although clearly the culprit was environmental. Researchers wondered whether some feature of Western lifestyle could be reducing the amount and diversity of microbes finding their way into infant digestive systems. If so, that diminished exposure could in turn diminish the activation of Th1, the key immune component in establishing healthy responses to foreign substances. As we've already discussed, when certain bacteria colonize the gut microbiome, the risk of food allergy increases. A group of Swedish researchers noticed that the guts of infants in Estonia had up to a thousandfold more bacteria that research suggests are beneficial than the guts of Swedish babies. And whereas allergy rates were low in Estonia, they were high in Sweden.

The correlation between allergy and the human microbiome may begin at birth. Several studies have found that allergic and nonallergic infants have different gut flora. In one Swedish study, children with food allergy had higher amounts of a bacterial species known as *Staphylococcus aureus* and lower amounts of *Bacteroides* and bifidobacteria, two other types. In a study from 2001, children with food allergy again had lower amounts of *Bacteroides* and bifidobacteria throughout their first year of life. Another investigation found that *Clostridium difficile* bacteria existed in greater numbers in the guts of allergic 12-month-olds.

That same year, a Finnish study probed even deeper. The researchers wanted to know if differences in the composition of gut flora in infants preceded the onset of allergies to egg and milk, along with other forms of atopy. They collected stool samples from 76 infants at 3 weeks of age and again at 3 months. All of the infants were born to families with a history of allergic diseases. Again, children with allergies had lower counts of bifidobacteria and higher counts of *C. difficile* than children without allergies. But another result was entirely new. "Neonatal intestinal microflora changes precede the development of atopic sensitization during infancy," the authors wrote. In other words, the differences in gut flora arose before the allergy. That meant that variations in the gut microbiome may do more than correlate with food allergy—they could actually cause it. A major Dutch study from 2007 looking at 957 infants at 1 month of age and again at 2 years demonstrated the same phenomenon.

What does all this have to do with birth by C-section? In the many studies unpacking the links between gut flora and allergy, two types—*Bacteroides* and bifidobacteria—pop up again and again. The more of these bacteria colonizing the gut, the less likely a child is to have an allergic disease. *C. difficile* (bacteria often associated with hospital-borne illnesses) also makes frequent appearances in the scientific literature, for the opposite reason—more *C. diff* equals more allergy. And it turns out that infants born by cesarean are more likely to have gut microbiomes with this exact profile: fewer *Bacteroides*, fewer bifidobacteria, and more *C. difficile*. By contrast, infants born vaginally are colonized exactly in reverse.

The exact mechanics driving the colonizing of a newborn's gut are controversial. Many digestive disease researchers have theorized that newborns become "seeded" with bacteria as they pass through the birth canal, a phenomenon dubbed "bacterial baptism." At this moment, emerging from the sealed-off world of the womb for the first time, infants ingest bacteria colonizing the mucosal tissue lining their pathway into the world. Babies born through C-section don't travel this route and so don't meet the wealth of microbes gathered there. It's this difference, the theory goes, that accounts, at least in part, for the escalated rates of immune-related diseases such as asthma, allergies, and inflammatory bowel disease. Studies have also tied the absence of bacterial baptism to obesity and several mental health conditions.

The evidence behind this theory is shaky. If the birth canal is responsible for the differences in gut flora seen between C-section and vaginal delivery babies, then those differences should be apparent immediately following birth. But studies have found that these variations aren't apparent until several days later. One study of stool samples showed no notable differences until five days after birth. And analyses of meconium—the very first stool sample an infant passes—have also found no meaningful disparities between the two groups. Other work has reported just the opposite. In a 2014 study, researchers at the University of Florida named four specific types of bacteria that differed in the meconium of infants born by C-section and those born vaginally. And in 2018, a group from China reported that infants delivered vaginally had more diverse microbiomes than those delivered by cesarean. They also found differences in the species colonizing the babies' guts.

But differences develop shortly after birth that may last for weeks or months. In one study of 98 infants, the 15 babies born via C-section had fewer *Bacteroides* and *Parabacteroides* species at four days and four months and more *Clostridium* species at one year compared to those born vaginally. In another 2017 study, an international group of researchers concluded that the stools of infants born by C-section had flora that were comparatively more similar to the bacteria colonizing their mothers' skin, as opposed to infants born vaginally. They also found that only infants who had passed through the birth canal and been breastfed had gut microbiomes plentiful in bifidobacteria, a large group of bacteria linked to health benefits including preventing colorectal cancer, treating some gastrointestinal disorders, and easing the symptoms of inflammatory bowel disease.

Thus far, most of the evidence leans away from delivery mode as a major shaper of the infant microbiome, yet there are enough data out there that the theory cannot be dismissed. And other factors may play a role, such as increased use of antibiotics for infants born via

C-section and the different microbes that babies born by each route may encounter during and following delivery at a hospital. Women who give birth via C-section may not go into labor, a process that often exposes the fetus to maternal bacteria by tearing infant membranes. At least one study reported that babies delivered by elective C-section, which typically avoids labor, have different microbiota compared to babies delivered by emergency C-section during labor. Whether or not a new mother breastfeeds will shape an infant's gut flora, and whether the mother has obesity could also have an effect.

In response to the notion that C-sections may leave infants without the benefit of scooping up some good maternal bacteria as they exit the womb, researchers from the United States and Puerto Rico tried an experimental remedy with eighteen mothers and their infants. Shortly before their scheduled C-sections, four of the eleven mothers who delivered by C-section inserted a folded piece of gauze into their vaginas for about an hour. The gauze was removed just before the delivery procedure and kept in a sterile environment. About a minute after delivery, the infant was swabbed with the gauze on the lips, face, chest, arms, legs, and the rest of the body for a total of about fifteen seconds. The researchers reported that during the first week of life, the swabbed infants had microbiomes resembling those of the seven infants born vaginally. The seven infants born by C-section and who were *not* swabbed had gut flora that was different from the other two groups.

Thus the concept of "vaginal seeding" was born. With this increasingly popular practice, infants born by cesarean have a cotton swab with vaginal fluid run over their lips, their face, and other areas.

As of now, no evidence exists that vaginal seeding is beneficial in preventing food allergy or any other disease associated with the microbiome. It's important to note that the study that launched the practice was far from ideal. Mothers who delivered by C-section had all received antibiotics prior to giving birth, whereas only one of the mothers delivering vaginally had antibiotics. None of the C-section mothers had gone into labor. Maternal obesity and pregnancy weight gain were also not factored into the results. And in this small group of infants, the differences between their microbiomes were slight and perhaps not as distinct as the study conclusion portrayed.

Vaginal seeding is risky because it could easily transfer dangerous viruses and fungi to the infant. The American College of Obstetricians and Gynecologists has declared that the practice should be done only in the context of an experimental study until we have more data on its safety and benefit. Parents who are considering vaginal seeding following a cesarean birth should speak with their doctors about it.

We have enough data to know that gut flora differs between infants born by C-section and those born vaginally, at least for a period of time. It also appears that these differences fade after not too long, especially after nursing is finished. Let's be clear: Mothers who had C-sections should not blame themselves for their child's food allergy. There is no evidence that this delivery route causes the condition on its own. Cesarean delivery is more likely part of a cluster of factors that together raise the risk of food allergy. C-sections are lifesaving procedures for many women and their newborns, and there should not be any guilt attached to having one. Today's mothers already face enough pressure and judgment without adding one more issue to the mix. Food allergy is no one's fault.

Still, the initial composition of the gut flora could have lasting health impacts that include increasing the risk of food allergy. We'll need more and larger studies to fully understand exactly why and how it factors into the likelihood of an infant's developing food allergy. Parents who are concerned that their future child may be at high risk for food allergy due to family history should speak with their obstetricians and allergists about how a C-section delivery may play into that risk and what to do about it.

COMMON CONCERNS ABOUT PREGNANCY, MATERNITY, AND FOOD ALLERGY

THE QUESTION	WHAT WE KNOW	HOW STRONG IS THE EVIDENCE?
Can the diet during pregnancy trigger food allergy in the developing infant?	No. Mom can eat anything she wants during pregnancy.	Very strong.
Is cesarean section delivery a risk factor for food allergy?	Possibly. Delivery by C-section may increase the risk of food allergy slightly, but not for everyone who has had this procedure.	Medium. Some articles have found evidence for this link; others have not.
Does a mother's diet during breastfeeding increase the likelihood of food allergy in a nursing infant?	No. Breastfeeding moms can eat anything they want.	Very strong. In fact, a 2014 study found that the rate of infant allergy to peanuts and tree nuts was lower among nonallergic mothers who ate these foods during lactation.
Do some types of formula increase the risk of food allergy?	No. There is no connection between formula and food allergy. Hydrolyzed and elemental formulas do not seem to prevent food allergy.	Very strong.

WHAT ELSE MATTERS?

As this chapter has illustrated so far, food allergy is likely the result of a cluster of factors, both environmental and genetic. Children with a food-allergic parent may develop the same allergy or they may not. Two children facing the same life circumstances may have very different experiences with food allergy. One child with nuclear family members allergic to peanuts who was delivered by C-section and raised in a sterile home may develop peanut allergy while another child with the same situation doesn't. And the population of people living with food allergy is a diverse bunch. The severity varies, the age of onset varies, and which foods are problematic varies.

Gradually, science is building a matrix of understanding about food allergy, laying out all the possible risk factors and the many ways in which the condition expresses itself. Researchers are also trying to identify the mechanisms that let our immune systems tolerate an allergen in the first place. Along with environment-based theories, genetics, and birth route, research has identified some other interesting, sometimes surprising influences.

Expectant parents may worry not only about the mode of delivery but also the timing. Since premature birth is often associated with health risks, it's reasonable to wonder whether an early arrival could make a child more susceptible to food allergy.

The evidence thus far shows that premature birth is not a risk factor. In fact, it may be just the opposite. A 2001 Finnish study of 72 premature babies and 65 full-term babies found that by age 10, the early birth group had half as much atopic disease as the other group. A few years later, a group from Canada tackled the same issue by looking at food allergy rates among 13,980 children born in 1995. Prematurity had no link to food allergy. Low birth weight was also irrelevant.

For families coping with a new diagnosis, it may also help to know that children may outgrow their food allergy. A study by David Fleischer at the University of Colorado found that people with peanut allergy had a 50 percent chance that the condition would disappear. Other studies have reported rates closer to 20 percent. Predicting which children may outgrow their allergies is currently not possible. However, we do know that many children who are allergic to eggs early in life are later able to tolerate cooked eggs. Children who eat baked goods containing eggs and dairy may be more likely to outgrow these allergies without any intervention, though it's not common and there's no guarantee. No one diagnosed with food allergy should ever just try a bit of the allergen to see if it's no longer a threat. For people who develop food allergy as adults, the immune system is unlikely to overcome the condition without medical intervention. Food allergy may also recur after it appears to have faded away.

In later chapters, we will introduce safe and proven methods for preventing and treating food allergy. Based on extensive evidence and bolstered by hundreds of success stories, our program for reversing food allergy will change the future of your or your child's condition from one you may have feared to one you will embrace.

THE BOTTOM LINE

- Children with parents who have food allergies are more likely to develop the condition, but many people with food allergy (diagnosed as adults or children) have no family history.

- No single gene has been identified as responsible for food allergy. Most likely, a combination of genes and/or environmental influences are responsible.

- Our surrounding environment may trigger changes to genes that can contribute to food allergy.

- There is no evidence that maternal diet during pregnancy and breastfeeding influences the risk of food allergy in infants.

- Some evidence suggests that delivery by cesarean section may increase the risk of food allergy, but if you have a C-section, this does not mean that your child will develop a food allergy.

Chapter 4

WHAT HAPPENS NOW? FOOD LABELS, KITCHENS, SCHOOLS, AND OTHER ESSENTIALS

*What to do, what to ask, and what to
learn following a food allergy diagnosis*

Leah and Hector Cuellar took a proactive approach to their parental allergy paranoia. When their son, William, was 4 months old, Leah fed him some peanut butter. Then she watched. When he turned red around his mouth and throat, she rushed to a nearby urgent care facility for an epinephrine shot. Further testing confirmed that William was allergic to peanuts. Also tree nuts and dairy.

They knew the logical next step was to purge their pantry of all things nuts. But as William grew from baby to toddler, the Cuellars tried something different. They kept their cabinets as they were. "He needs to learn to be around them," says Leah. Instead of banishing nuts from his reach, they are teaching William, now 5, to ask if a food is safe.

That hasn't made life risk-free. At Easter when William was 4, Leah asked her mother to keep the candy and desserts nut-free. "So she bought Peanut M&M's," recalls Leah. When William was younger, his mother or father had to be with him at all times—especially after he tried to eat a Nutter Butter he found at the playground when he was 18 months old. They chose a preschool with a no-nut policy and trained the staff to inject epinephrine. And they worry constantly about their well-meaning relatives who don't understand food allergy. "We tell them," says Leah, "and they don't get it."

FIRST MOVES

This chapter provides a step-by-step guide for moving forward. Families don't need to do everything at once. Parents of toddlers with food allergy don't need to wonder how your children will handle life on their own as a first priority. But little by little, living with food allergy will become a manageable reality, albeit with a few necessary changes.

Chapter 7 will introduce our program for reversing food allergy. But even families who are ready to march into this new era will need to stop at home first. And the kitchen is the first place that needs to be made safe.

Pantry and Refrigerator

Many parents will opt to keep certain allergens out of their home entirely. It's easy enough for an unsupervised toddler with a milk allergy to grab a carton from the fridge when no one is looking. The same goes for packages of peanuts or tree nuts that are harmless snacks for most people. And keeping the refrigerator and pantry clear of the allergen itself is a simple way to eliminate the risk. If you're worried about your milk-allergic child drinking milk at home, then don't have it in your home.

But some families want to keep allergens in the house for non-allergic members. A nonallergic sibling who loves peanut butter won't readily give it up for a younger brother or sister diagnosed with a peanut allergy—and many parents won't want to give up the beautiful convenience of a PB&J lunch for a child happy with one. Eliminating milk might change your morning coffee routine. Weekend omelets aren't possible for families who stop buying eggs on account of an egg-allergic child.

There are alternatives when it isn't practical or desirable for families to banish allergens from the home. Dried goods—nuts, nut butters, snack foods that contain dairy or eggs—can be kept in high cabinets away from a toddler's reach. Dangerous refrigerated items can be moved toward the back or into a drawer or even a separate container. As allergic babies grow into allergic children, restrictions are easier to explain. Color-coded stickers can help children identify foods that are safe for them. Food-allergic children could have their own space in the pantry filled with safe-to-consume snacks.

Many families initially banish the allergen from their homes following the diagnosis but gradually make adjustments. One mother put nuts and seeds in plastic containers on a shelf so high that an adult would need a stepstool to reach it. She also gave her son his own snack drawer. Another family learned to live without nuts even when the food-allergic child was old enough to avoid them at home. Occasionally the family treated themselves to a PB&J sandwich outside of the house when the food-allergic child wasn't around. Instead of a safe space in the kitchen, one family has a "not safe" space, where they keep individually wrapped snacks containing allergens.

Cooking

A food allergy diagnosis also brings new rules for cooking. Cutting boards, pots, pans, and knives used for cooking must be thoroughly cleaned. It may be best to keep a cutting board that allergens never come in contact with. For severely allergic children, families may wish to purchase a set of pots and pans that are used to prepare allergen-free food only. Countertops and cooking surfaces, including grills, should be cleaned thoroughly if an allergen has been placed there. Utensils should be cleaned after stirring or chopping anything containing an allergen. Cooks should wash their hands thoroughly after handling an allergen.

Depending on the meal, food-allergic children may want to stay out of the kitchen during food prep. A child with a wheat allergy shouldn't hang around the kitchen while you're making bread or baking a cake because the flour is easily airborne. Many families with wheat-allergic members may opt for a wheat-free kitchen. Matthew Friend's family, however, took a different approach. Matthew was diagnosed with a severe wheat allergy in 1999, when he was 9 months old. "I was fed baby cereal and I blew up into hives," he says. Even skin contact could trigger a reaction. The gluten-free cupcakes his mother baked for him to bring to birthday parties when he was growing up in Chicago were the envy of his friends. But his parents opted to not banish wheat from the house. He ate gluten-free pasta at dinners where his siblings had wheat pasta. Years later, he says that decision gave him a good foundation for life as an adult. "The rest of the world is not going to cater to you," he says. "You have to be prepared to live in the real world."

Cross-Contact

Protecting a food-allergic child or adult from a reaction is often an eye-opening experience. To see the world through their eyes is to see danger where the rest of us see pleasure—or at the very least nothing harmful. A child who dislikes cheese can take it off the burger without consequence. A child allergic to cow dairy cannot eat a hamburger even touched by cheese.

Cross-contact occurs when an allergen touches another food. A bit of peanut butter on a piece of bread; a drop of milk from a spilled glass hitting the scrambled eggs; a spoon that served shrimp salad then used for the macaroni. The proteins that trigger immune systems to react rub off easily, leaving invisible but very real traces behind.

Unfortunately, the genuine threat of cross-contact means parents must be vigilant. Food-allergic children usually can't be left to get food on their own at a party or a hotel buffet. Parents may feel uncomfortable sending back a restaurant meal with accidental cheese, but usually that's the only option. Soup ladles can't be safely moved from a dairy-containing pot to a nondairy pot. The spatula that flipped a grilled cheese can't be used to flip a dairy-allergic child's omelet, and the spatula that flipped an omelet can't be used to flip an egg-allergic child's burger. The knife that sliced the tofu can't be used to slice the chicken for a soy-allergic child.

This level of vigilance may sound exhausting—and it can be. But food-allergic families become accustomed to their requirements. They integrate safe cooking practices into their kitchen. They identify safe restaurants. They know when to stay watchful and when the coast is clear. A checklist such as the one below may help, especially during the early days following a diagnosis:

- Cabinets
  - Designate a shelf for safe products, perhaps giving food-allergic children their own space in the pantry.
  - Move risky household essentials to higher cabinets out of toddler reach.
- Refrigerator
  - Consider eliminating allergens from the home temporarily or permanently.
  - Label unsafe foods with warning stickers or keep them in a separate container.
- Cooking
  - Clean counters, knives, and all cooking equipment thoroughly with warm, soapy water; don't depend on wiping to remove dangerous food proteins.
  - Consider separate cooking equipment for severely allergic children.
  - Avoid using the same cooking utensils in allergen and nonallergen dishes.
  - Consider preparing the food-allergic child's meal first.

- Dining table
  - Do not allow food-allergic children to consume food that has come in contact with their allergen.
  - Watch for spills or other exposure.
  - Keep safe serving utensils and dishes far from those in contact with food allergens.

Where Allergens Are Hiding in Your Home

Sometimes food allergens are lurking in unsuspected places. When scouring your home, be sure to look at the labels of these items (along with any new household products you may purchase after your initial search):

- Gelatin
- Pectin
- Emulsifiers. These substances, which help oil and water stay together, may contain egg or dairy.
- Food-based oils. Although most cooking oils contain no protein (which is the allergenic part of a food), some do. Because people with food allergies may react to even a minute amount of the protein, we recommend avoiding oils with your allergen, especially when dining outside the home.
- Toothpaste. Some contain dairy.
- Drugs. Check for milk powder listed among the inert ingredients, for example.
- Plant-based cleaning solutions or oils
- Cosmetics
- Creams/lotions

The food allergy advocacy organization Food Allergy Research & Education (FARE) has a useful list of questions for families who aren't sure whether to remove allergens from their home or try another approach. These questions may be useful to consider as you make changes to your family's lifestyle following a diagnosis:

- What has your experience been with reactions and accidental exposure?

- If you were to remove problem foods, how difficult would this be for other family members?

- How many children are at home? If a child has food allergies, how old are they and how much responsibility do they normally take for managing the food they eat?

- If you decide it is best to eliminate allergen-containing foods at home, how will you help your child with food allergies learn how to manage outside the home when contact with allergens is possible?

- If you decide not to eliminate allergen-containing foods at home, how will you teach your child with food allergies about which foods are safe and unsafe?

As you ask these questions, it may be useful to remember that your answers may change over time. Just as is true for nonallergic children, a toddler's needs are different from a teenager's needs. New arrangements will arise over the years. The sighs of relief will come. And your children *will* learn to take care of themselves.

UNDERSTANDING FOOD LABELS

Ridding your home of potential food threats and ensuring that only allergy-safe products are tossed into the grocery cart require an intimate relationship with food labeling. Even food shoppers untouched by food allergy are familiar with the lingo: *may contain peanuts; prepared in a facility that also handles tree nuts.* Whether these messages indicate a product to avoid or a company protecting itself isn't always—if ever—clear.

Understanding the origin of these disclosures is a useful place to start. Once upon a time, of course, there were no processed foods and people didn't have to wonder about what they were eating because it was obvious. The first time the government stepped in to regulate food labeling was 1906, when President Theodore Roosevelt passed the Pure Food and Drug Act, also known as the Wiley Act (named after the USDA's chief chemist, Harvey Washington Wiley, who finally persuaded the government that such a law was needed by feeding a group of young men increasing amounts of formaldehyde and other preservatives in order to demonstrate their lethality). The Food and Drug Administration (FDA) already existed, but the Wiley Act marks its functional start.

The Fair Packaging and Labeling Act, passed in 1966, required that ingredients be listed on all food products. The Nutrition Labeling and Education Act came next, in 1990. That act is why we have nutrition labels on packaged foods. It also brought to light simmering issues about food allergy—namely, that companies could not presume any allergen to be present in "insignificant levels" because even the tiniest amount could trigger a reaction. All allergens, the agency declared, should be voluntarily listed on labels. Simply noting that a product "may contain" this or that allergen was not enough.

In the late 1990s, officials at the FDA noticed an uptick in product recalls. Repeated alerts from snack manufacturers about undisclosed egg and peanut in their products led these officials to wonder just how widespread the problem was. How often were food-allergic people unknowingly exposed to hazardous ingredients? They knew the answer could mean taking action to protect the American public from food allergens, something the FDA had never had to consider before.

Investigators from the FDA headed to Minnesota and Wisconsin. Between September 1999 and March 2000, they checked samples of cookies, ice cream, and various other snack foods made by a randomly selected 85 companies. They were looking for products that contained undeclared peanut or egg. The results were disheartening. "Some 25% of the companies failed to list all ingredients on their products, and about half did not check the labels to make sure that all ingredients used in a product were listed on the product label," read a news report in *BMJ* (formerly *British Medical Journal*). Many products had become contaminated with other food allergens during the manufacturing process without anyone knowing. And only half of the companies compared the labels and ingredients to make sure that everything that should be listed was listed.

At the time of the report's completion in 2001, the FDA was requiring food manufacturers to declare all ingredients except natural ones that existed in just trace amounts. But in light of the FDA's findings, clearly that wasn't enough. And individual states were simultaneously recognizing the need for more stringent regulation where food allergens were concerned. In addition to ingredients missing from labels and potential allergens inadvertently finding their way into foods, the food-allergic community also faced the challenge of terminology. Milk protein in processed foods could go by many other names—casein, caseinates, lactose, whey. A product labeled as nondairy could contain milk by-products. Not every family with an egg-allergic member would know to avoid albumin. The term *natural flavor* could be hiding food allergens. And companies might not disclose what the food manufacturing industry referred to as "incidental additives," substances present in such tiny levels as to be almost undetectable—though not necessarily to the immune system of an allergic person. "To avoid a major allergen, a food-allergic consumer would need to call the manufacturer before purchasing the product to confirm that an allergen was present," noted a 2001 article in *FDA Consumer*, an FDA publication.

That brings us to the Food Allergen Labeling and Consumer Protection Act of 2004, better known as FALCPA. This act required packaged food manufacturers to adhere to stricter labeling requirements beginning in 2006. According to FALCPA, the presence of the eight most common allergens must be indicated in the list of ingredients or next to the ingredients, following the word *contains.* The act also required the use of plain English, so any unfamiliar term would be followed by its recognizable name—for example, "lecithin (soy)."

But FALCPA falls short in several ways. The most glaringly obvious issue is that the act covers only the eight most common allergens, even though more than a hundred have been identified. Sesame seeds aren't covered by FALCPA, for example, even though the allergy to sesame likely affects more than a million people in the United States, making it the ninth most common food allergen. In Canada, sesame allergy rivals peanut for accidental exposure. And Canada and many other countries require packaged food companies to disclose the sesame in their ingredient lists. Less common but still concerning allergens include corn, meat, gelatin, other seeds (sunflower, poppy), mustard, and garlic, among others.

There are plenty of products that FALCPA doesn't cover. The makers of prescription and over-the-counter drugs aren't required to list allergens on their packaging. Kosher foods also fall outside of the FALCPA umbrella. So do personal care items, restaurant foods in wrappers or containers, and alcoholic drinks, such as mixers, which aren't regulated by the FDA. (FALCPA also doesn't require agriculture sellers to label their fruits and vegetables, probably because it sensibly trusts the public to know that apples contain, well, apple. And it doesn't have purview over pesticides and other chemicals added to produce.)

Also, FALCPA doesn't regulate use of the term *may contain,* which means manufacturers are free to use it even though it's meaningless. Think about it this way: If a box of cookies carries a warning that reads "may contain milk," that could mean any number of things. Maybe the cookies were made on the same factory line as a milk-containing product. If so, was it made on the same day? Was it made on a different day? Was the machinery cleaned in between? Does the company ever clean the factory line? Could dust from another line make it over to the cookie line? Does the company test for allergens? If so, what threshold levels is it monitoring? Does this *may contain* sentence actually mean anything?

All of this can lead to many confusing hours spent trying to parse the words on the side of a box of cookies. Kim and Dave Friedman, whose daughter was allergic to tree nuts, remember endless phone calls to companies asking about whether one product or another was safe to keep in their home. Trips to the supermarket became stressful endeavors to find clear information. One store told her that the only way to be sure an item from their in-house brand was free from allergens was to send her the UPC code from the packaging—and to do this every time they shopped because the factory periodically makes changes. "Who would have thought that ketchup would be made on a factory line that also handles cashews?" says Kim.

Some manufacturers add language that begins "This product was processed on machinery that processes nuts" or "We are unable to guarantee . . ." Yet the FDA has no guidelines for measuring cross-contamination or for these types of advisory labels. At the root of this problem is the fact that the FDA does not have a clear way of measuring the lowest level of an allergen that will cause a reaction, known as the allergen threshold. The agency has said that there aren't enough data available to set these thresholds. But without them, food manufacturers have no way to know whether the risk of cross-contamination in their factory ever leads to actual cross-contamination of their products. The result is a frustrating one for people with food allergies. As one legal review of FALCPA puts it: "Companies are instead incentivized to be overinclusive on their advisory labels, while remaining unmotivated to transform their practices to avoid cross-contact." And *may contain* statements are entirely voluntarily, so consumers should not consider them a substitute for reading the ingredient list. As Sharon Chinthrajah, who directs the clinical research program at Stanford, puts it, "Labeling laws do not protect an individual."

There are other, subtler concerns with FALCPA. Highly refined oils do not need to be disclosed according to the law, and technically such oils should not contain proteins. It's the proteins that are the problem when it comes to immune system attacks. But some people with food allergy react to highly refined oils because they may still contain enough protein to cause a reaction, making their omission from FALCPA requirements a problem. The rules may also carry disincentives for manufacturers. Tree nuts, crustaceans, and fish—three of the top eight allergens—are not single items but groups of foods, even though a person may be allergic to only one or some of the species included in the category. Not everyone who is allergic to almonds is allergic to hazelnuts, and not everyone allergic to mussels is allergic to shrimp. But foods aren't labeled according to what species is present, only by the broader category. As a result, people in no danger of reacting to a particular packaged food may still stay away from it.

Finally, FALCPA leaves some room for exemptions. A company can notify the FDA that a particular ingredient "does not contain an allergenic protein" or petition for an exemption to FALCPA labeling requirements if the company believes that an ingredient "does not cause an allergic response that poses risk to human health."

But the exemption clause leaves much room for error. Reviews of notifications focus on examining whether the protein in question binds with IgE, the telltale indicator that the body will suffer a food reaction. To grant a petition, on the other hand, the FDA needs to be sure that the threatening protein exists in amounts below the allergen threshold. Both of these conditions can be slippery. In the notifications filed to date, ingredient descriptions weren't always clear, making it hard to determine that a product didn't contain a particular allergenic protein. Some submissions included the original form of the ingredient but not its identity in the available product. That can be problematic because sometimes the chemistry changes en route from raw ingredient to packaged snack. Companies weren't always clear about the manufacturing process.

Some exemption petitions used irrelevant guidelines for insisting that their product satisfied the allergen threshold. For example, some companies called their foods "hypoallergenic" using a guideline for formula set by the American Academy of Pediatrics. These guidelines don't even guarantee that infants allergic to milk won't react to formula, and they certainly can't be broadly applied to snack foods. Some companies insisted that the allergenic protein had been rendered harmless by the manufacturing process, but offered no evidence. In other words, the exemption process is hardly foolproof, and companies trying to game the system could find a way to do so. That being said, as of July 2018, the FDA has received just eight notifications and four petitions. And companies willing to take the risk of harming a food-allergic consumer are the exception, not the rule. As imperfect as they may be, labels are the single most reliable source for avoiding allergens lurking in processed foods.

Most recently, the FDA Food Safety Modernization Act, enacted in 2011, has attempted to safeguard the public from food-related dangers. Included in this act is a requirement for companies to create a "food allergen control plan" in order to minimize or prevent these substances in products, monitor the effectiveness of whatever controls are put in place, and take corrective action should any allergens slip through.

In 2014, the European Union passed a new law requiring companies to list allergens clearly and legibly and restaurants and cafés to provide allergen information. Food Standards Australia New Zealand has required companies in those countries to disclose ten allergens on package labels since 1991; however, vague language has the agency considering improvements in terminology, such as not lumping mollusks in with fish and crustaceans, defining tree nuts, and differentiating between cereals linked to wheat allergy and those linked to gluten intolerance. Canada, by contrast, requires companies to list nine tree nuts by specific name, the name of the fish (rather than its broader category), and the source of the wheat allergen and/or gluten.

Regarding medications, the MMR (measles, mumps, rubella) and influenza vaccines are safe for egg-allergic children and adults, including those with previous episodes of anaphylaxis. However, it is best to alert the healthcare professional administering the vaccine about an egg allergy beforehand. Medications contained in gel caps, which are made of gelatin, are not safe for people with gelatin allergy.

THRESHOLDS AND ANAPHYLAXIS

People with food allergy often wonder how much is too much. Will even trace amounts of an allergen trigger a reaction? For most individuals, it takes about 300 milligrams or more to set off the immune system—that's about the equivalent of a single nut, a teaspoon of milk, or one tenth of a shrimp. But sometimes the threshold is lower and even an accidental touch can trigger a reaction (allergic reactions almost always occur within the first two hours of exposure). Allergy thresholds can vary person to person and throughout a life; exercise, sleep, illness, stress, puberty, and even altitude can alter the amount of allergen your body can tolerate. For this reason, people with food allergies can never let their guard down.

The word *anaphylaxis* strikes fear into the heart of anyone who has seen a child—body swollen and red, breathing labored—rushed to the emergency room, or who has been through this ordeal personally. The term, which means "without protection" in Greek, is often wrongly used to refer to fatal or nearly fatal allergic reactions. What anaphylaxis really refers to is a reaction involving two or more areas of the body—say, both hives on the arms and an itchy throat. Anaphylaxis becomes dangerous when the internal organs begin reacting—marked by difficulty breathing, wheezing, a drop in blood pressure, or vomiting, for example. Epinephrine is the first critical step for treating severe anaphylaxis; antihistamines and steroids should both be used only after epinephrine, for a severe anaphylactic reaction.

INTRODUCING EPINEPHRINE

Epinephrine is one of the first new vocabulary words for any family with a food allergy diagnosis. The word is synonymous with adrenaline, the first hormone ever discovered. The drug form of epinephrine, prescribed for a wide range of allergies, has saved countless lives.

Back in 1859, a British doctor named Henry Salter made a peculiar observation: asthma, he noticed, could be cured by "sudden alarm or violent fleeting excitements." That description calls to mind the phrase most closely associated with the adrenal glands: *fight or flight*. In an emergency situation, it's the rush of adrenaline that gives us the power to slay or flee an enemy.

The discovery of epinephrine, which can refer to both natural adrenaline and also the synthesized drug, stems from a long history. Eustachius, an Italian considered a founder of the science of human anatomy, documented the existence of the adrenal glands in 1552. Scientists across Europe uncovered their exact structure over the next three hundred years. But although they figured out that the glands contained an extract, they didn't know what that extract did.

In the late nineteenth century, a British physician named George Oliver solved the mystery using adrenal glands obtained from his local butcher in the small spa town where he lived. He saw the powerful effect the glands had. "The effect upon the blood vessels is to cause extreme contraction of arteries," he wrote, "so that the blood pressure is enormously raised." In one experiment, Oliver injected his son with some extract from the adrenal glands he'd procured and watched how it constricted the child's blood vessels. A disbelieving colleague of his, Edward Schäfer, agreed to do the same on a dog in his own laboratory and confirmed that his friend was not as crazy as he'd first assumed. The tool Schäfer used to measure blood pressure quickly reached its upper limit. They'd discovered the incredible effect that adrenaline has on the body.

Within a few years, Jokichi Takamine, a Japanese American biochemist who favored a bicycle mustache and bottle glasses, created synthetic adrenaline, patented it, and sold the patent to a pharmaceutical company. (Takamine also brought Washington, D.C., its first cherry trees by arranging them as a gift from the mayor of Tokyo.) Initially called adrenaline, the product was soon renamed epinephrine. Hailed as a bit of a miracle drug at first, epinephrine was once used to treat bubonic plague and bedwetting before finding its proper place as a lifesaver for people with asthma and allergies. (The drug is also used during certain types of surgery.)

Biologically, natural adrenaline works by attaching itself to adrenergic receptors, proteins that sit on the outside of many cells in the body. This binding activates the sympathetic nervous system, which launches the flight-or-fight response. Our pupils dilate, our heart rate increases, our blood redirects its flow from nonessential organs to skeletal muscle. We become pumped, energized for a challenge— suddenly able to run for our lives, lift a car off a child, or defeat whatever Goliath we are facing—that our normal state would not allow.

Epinephrine also counteracts the reactions of anaphylaxis. During an allergic reaction, blood vessels constrict, as if attempting to stop the passage of poison through the body. Blood pressure plummets. Rarely the airways may tighten, making breathing extremely difficult. In a severe reaction, all of this occurs within minutes. Epinephrine reverses this course, relaxing the smooth muscle lining the airways and raising blood pressure. Redness, inflammation, and hives can also dissipate as this synthetic adrenaline winds its way through the body. Crucially, the drug also widens the airways.

When a self-injector was invented in the 1970s, it was initially given to soldiers to protect themselves against chemical warfare. Soon enough, though, researchers realized that the drug combined with the auto-injector device were ideal for treating allergic reactions. The FDA approved the first brand-name product, the EpiPen, in 1987. The first indication was asthma, as if answering a call buried in Henry Salter's 1859 observation that sudden excitement stopped asthma attacks. What he'd seen was adrenaline at work, though he couldn't have known it at the time. The product soon found a ready home among people with food allergy and quickly became an indispensable companion for families coping with these diagnoses.

How to Use Epinephrine

Epinephrine is the drug of choice for anaphylaxis, according to the World Allergy Organization. Anyone diagnosed with a food allergy should be carrying at least two epinephrine self-injectors at all times—we recommend two in case the first one doesn't take effect quickly enough. The prescription should be kept up to date and the dosage should be confirmed as appropriate for the weight of the patient every time the prescription is refilled. But integrating the self-injector into daily life isn't as easy or obvious as it may sound. Yet as Eric Graber-Lopez, whose son grew up with multiple food allergies, puts it, "What's the alternative? It's a lifesaving tool."

A word before diving into the evidence-based how-tos of epinephrine. The studies of this medication often focus on its ability to prevent allergy-related severe reactions or deaths (which are *very* rare). Thus many of the studies involve statistics on fatalities. We encourage families not to be daunted by this measurement and instead use epinephrine when necessary. The risk of death is not always at stake when the body encounters a food allergen. In other words, we advise families to use the research to inform their decisions, not to send them into fits of panic.

FOOD ALLERGY SYMPTOMS AND TREATMENTS

SYMPTOM (WITHIN TWO HOURS OF INGESTING A FOOD)*	TREATMENT
Hives, runny nose, itchy mouth, itchy throat	H1 blockers (over-the-counter allergy medication, such as Zyrtec or Claritin); apply ice to skin or suck on ice to relieve oral symptoms.
Abdominal pain, cramps, vomiting	H2 blockers (also called H2 antagonists, such as Pepto Bismol, Zantac, or Pepcid) and/or H1 blockers. Swallowing ice water may also offer symptom relief. Do not use warm packs.
Hypotension, wheezing, dizziness, extensive vomiting	Epinephrine injectable device.
Headaches, bloating, gas	Consult physician. These symptoms are not typically associated with a food allergy and may be due to a different underlying condition.

*Wheat allergy symptoms may appear more than two hours after ingestion.

Epinephrine should be used for certain types of allergic reactions, though not for all of them. A large percentage of food-related reactions are mild. Hives often clear up without medication. Itchiness fades in short order. Redness disappears. But a mild reaction one year can easily be followed by a severe one the next, even to the same amount of allergen. According to a study of 48 food fatalities in the UK between 1999 and 2006, more than half occurred in people whose most recent allergic reaction had been so mild that a doctor might not have even prescribed epinephrine. Other reports say three of every four people who've died from food anaphylaxis had experienced only minor reactions previously. It's worth repeating: Fatal reactions happen but are extremely rare.

Most deaths due to anaphylaxis occur because someone outside of a medical facility didn't use injectable epinephrine soon enough. In a study of six fatal and seven nonfatal cases of childhood anaphylaxis resulting from a food allergy, none of the children who died received epinephrine before their airways began to close. And in a review of sixty-three U.S. deaths due to food anaphylaxis, only seven had auto-injectors on hand at the time of the reaction. A study by Canadian immunologist Estelle Simons found that around 30 percent of prescriptions for self-injectors were never filled.

Many parents obtain their first epinephrine device with no idea how to use it. Although pharmacies provide written instructions when prescriptions are filled, few parents receive any kind of direct in-person training. But even though most parents say they feel confident about using the injector, that's often not true at the moment of need. In a 2006 review of 601 cases of anaphylaxis in the United States, researchers at the University of Tennessee identified the need for more effective teaching on the use of epinephrine. Sometimes preparation is the shortfall. One survey found that in nearly half of sixty-eight cases of food-related anaphylaxis, patients did not have epinephrine with them even though they'd suffered an attack from exactly the same food before. Granted, that particular study is from twenty-five years ago, and families today are far more aware of the perils of food allergens lurking in every restaurant dish and packaged food. Yet the lesson still applies: *if you or your child have food allergy, carry epinephrine.*

A 2006 study found that for 122 UK children with food allergy, nearly 70 percent of parents could not use the auto-injector, didn't have one, or didn't know when to use it. The problem continues into adulthood: A U.S. survey of 1,000 adults who'd had a severe anaphylactic reaction found that half of those who'd had two prior allergy attacks did not have an epinephrine prescription. The burden of mishaps isn't all on the patient. Sometimes even doctors prescribing an auto-injector don't know how to use it. Or they fail to encourage families to seek training or help them arrange it. Having seen it demonstrated beforehand increased the chances of a parent using epinephrine appropriately by more than fourfold in the UK study. Parents who'd consulted with an allergy specialist (rather than a general practitioner) and those who'd obtained information from allergy advocacy groups were similarly better equipped. A study from 2016 looking at anxiety and quality of life among food allergy families found that having a solid partnership with healthcare professionals and equipping children to self-manage their condition would help families best adapt to the challenges of food allergy. And in a Montreal-based study of more than 1,200 children who required epinephrine prescriptions, more than half of parents feared they would hurt their child with an injection, use the medicine incorrectly, or cause a damaging side effect.

People with food allergy who are at the highest risk of a fatal reaction include those with asthma, teenagers (who often fail to carry epinephrine), and those who cannot afford the medication or have poor access to healthcare facilities. Education is central to preventing food allergy deaths. We have begun training programs in economically disadvantaged areas of Chicago, New York City, East Palo Alto, and San Francisco to ensure that those at highest risk know how and when to use epinephrine. We hope others will join us so that we can move forward as an inclusive food-allergy community.

As one immunologist put it: "Autoinjectors cannot save lives when they are used too late, misused, not carried, or when an inadequate dose is absorbed." That about sums it up.

Individuals and families coping with food allergy should consult with their allergists about the correct use of epinephrine. Anyone who may be responsible for injecting an allergy sufferer with the medication must know when to use it, where to inject it, and what to do after administering treatment. There is no substitute for in-person training. However, here are a few basics:

- Waiting too long (more than a few minutes after crucial symptoms appear) to administer medication is a chief contributor to food allergy fatalities.

- More serious reactions should trigger immediate epinephrine use: shortness of breath, coughing, a weak pulse, a tightened throat, difficulty breathing, light-headedness, or loss of consciousness.

- Sudden difficulty in breathing is an emergency. Epinephrine should be given right away and an ambulance should be called.

- Epinephrine should be injected into the side of the thigh only.

- The medication can cause side effects. People may feel their heart is racing. They may turn pale or develop a headache. They may feel nauseated. These symptoms will dissipate. The risk of serious problems resulting from epinephrine is extremely low and typically does not outweigh the risk of not providing the medication during an allergic reaction.

- **Always accompany the use of epinephrine with a call to 911.** Anyone with an allergic response strong enough to warrant the drug should be seen by a medical professional as soon as possible. The words to say to the emergency dispatcher are "severe, life-threatening anaphylaxis."

- It is ideal to have two auto-injectors available at all times. Some allergic reactions will require a second dose of the medication.

- Several products are now available: EpiPen, AUVI-Q, Adrenaclick, and generic epinephrine auto-injectors. Patients should speak with their allergists and insurance providers to determine which product is right for them. We strongly advise against using a homemade epinephrine kit.

- Epinephrine prescriptions should be replaced every year, confirming that the dosage is correct for the weight of the patient. However, patients should also know that the drug typically remains stable for about two years after its expiration date.

- Anyone diagnosed with a food allergy should have a reaction plan printed and readily available for anyone in the household, workplace, school, or after-school program to use. Those friends and relatives who visit frequently or who often have the patient in their homes should also have copies.

The Dos and Don'ts of Epinephrine Usage

Do have someone call 911 if you are having a severe allergic reaction and need epinephrine.

Don't wait for the reaction to worsen before seeking help.

Do give epinephrine immediately for severe allergic reactions. Epinephrine will not hurt a person even if it's given too soon, and it works best when given early in a reaction.

Don't wait too long. Epinephrine does not work as well during the later stages of an allergic reaction.

Do give epinephrine in the outer mid-thigh. Hold the injector against the thigh for ten seconds to deliver the medication.

Don't inject epinephrine any place other than the outer mid-thigh.

Do administer epinephrine when wheezing occurs as part of a food allergy reaction.

Don't give an inhaler when wheezing occurs as part of a food allergy reaction.

Do sit down and ask someone to get your epinephrine if you have it with you during an allergic reaction.

Don't run to get your epinephrine injector on your own; running increases the severity of an allergic reaction.

Do wait five minutes after injecting epinephrine before seeking further help. Signs that the medication has started working include shaky hands and a suddenly fast-beating heart.

Don't seek help immediately after injecting epinephrine. The medication takes about five minutes to work.

Do administer a second dose of epinephrine after five minutes if the allergic symptoms are not improving or the allergic individual is nonresponsive. If the medication is having an effect but some symptoms persist, it's safe to wait an additional five minutes before the second dose (ten minutes total between doses).

Don't delay giving a second dose if the allergic individual is non-responsive or symptoms are not improving.

Do keep two epinephrine injectors with you at all times. The medication should be stored at room temperature. Be aware of expiration dates and replace the prescription when necessary (usually annually).

Don't keep epinephrine in a hot car, in the refrigerator, or in a cooler with ice or ice packs.

Epinephrine at School

Eric Graber-Lopez recalls the challenge of integrating epinephrine into the daily life of his son, Sebastian, who was diagnosed with allergies to wheat, milk, and egg when he was 4 months old. He and his wife never left the house without the medication. Even when Sebastian was a toddler, they would show him that they were packing the epinephrine when they left the house. "It became like putting on his shoes," says Eric. As soon as Sebastian was old enough, he kept an auto-injector around his waist at all times (companies sell belts specifically for this purpose). "We strived to give him incremental control over his care as he got older," he says. Then came kindergarten. "Where it became tricky was at school," Eric recalls.

Most parents want to keep an epinephrine injector at school, and all schools these days accommodate that need. But schools follow a range of practices with storing the drug. Some allow students to keep their medication with them; others don't. At Sebastian's first school, the administrators wanted the prescription kept in the nurse's office. "That defeats the whole purpose," says Eric. In the event of an allergy attack, Sebastian would have to alert a teacher, who would in turn alert the nurse. By the time the injection reached Sebastian, it could easily be too late.

In Sebastian's case, persistence won the day. The school agreed to allow him to wear his epinephrine holster or, as he got older, keep the injector in his backpack or wherever was most convenient. Eric and his wife also met with teachers every year to review the instructions for how to handle an allergy attack and made sure to train the staff in using epinephrine themselves, even if they'd seen it demonstrated elsewhere.

As is true with many aspects of school, the parents of children with food allergy need to become advocates for their child's welfare. With food allergy rates being what they are, most academic institutions are familiar with concerns surrounding exposure. The School Access to Emergency Epinephrine Act, passed in 2013, provides support for states to enact policies that help protect students at risk of anaphylaxis, such as legal protection of trained professionals who administer epinephrine to treat an allergy attack. But that should not stop parents and students from taking whatever steps they need to feel confident that the school is equipped to provide whatever measures necessary, as soon as they become necessary, should a child experience a reaction.

We recommend that parents provide schools with two auto-injectors per child. We also recommend that schools agree that one student's epinephrine can be used for another student should the need arise. Parents should be aware that schools typically require that any auto-injectors have a shelf life of one year at the time it's provided.

Epinephrine Choices and Price Tags

It's impossible to leave the subject of epinephrine without discussing the cost. California-based mom Elizabeth Liptak, whose daughter, Amelia, has food allergy, sums up her experience incorporating epinephrine into her life in one word: "expensive." She purchases three two-injector packs per year—one for home, one for school, one for the car—because the medicine has a one-year expiration date. Most recently she paid $249 (after insurance coverage) for all three packs. But another year, the same purchase came to $900. Insurance typically covers some portion of the cost, but families will still shoulder a significant burden at the checkout counter.

In 2016, Mylan, the pharmaceutical company selling the brand name EpiPen, came under government scrutiny for raising the price of the auto-injector from about $50 to just over $600 over the course of about eight years. The hike left the company with about $1.1 billion in profits and also left many patients unable to afford the medication. The criticism that followed (and an appearance before the House Committee on Oversight and Reform) eventually led the company to cut the price in half. In August 2018, generic epinephrine finally became available. But although this entry to the market seems to have calmed the year-to-year price fluctuations, it hasn't necessarily made the drug cheaper—the initial generic price tag was $300. A new Illinois law requires insurance companies to cover epinephrine for anyone under age 18 starting in January 2020, the first legislation of this kind.

Meanwhile, another auto-injector, AUVI-Q, which first became available in 2013 but was taken off the market due to technical issues, returned to market in 2017. AUVI-Q is a smaller device—Eric Graber-Lopez says Sebastian, now a teenager, favors it because it fits in his pocket, which means no standing out among his friends for carrying around an injector the width of two Sharpie markers. "That was a life-changer," says Eric.

Families new to the world of food allergy will find the option that suits them best. Factored into the equation should be considerations of cost, stress, and ease of use. From a medical perspective, though, all that matters is having the epinephrine and knowing how and when to use it properly. For families unable to afford their prescription, your allergist may be able to help find resources for financial assistance. Every person living with food allergy should have a filled prescription for epinephrine—period.

ANTIHISTAMINES AND DIPHENHYDRAMINE

Epinephrine isn't always necessary. When an exposure results in mild symptoms—hives, abdominal pain, itchy or congested nose, watering eyes, swelling, itchy throat, or redness—then cetirizine (Zyrtec) or loratadine (Claritin) is a more appropriate response.

Applying ice can also help. We do not typically recommend diphen-hydramine (Benadryl) because it can cause sleepiness, low blood pressure, and heart arrhythmias.

The medical care of food allergy can be intimidating. Parents become understandably nervous. Children are often too young to take control. School staff may appear too busy to pay attention to the needs of a single child. But the basic measures required to protect someone diagnosed with food allergy are straightforward and readily integrated into daily life. "It's a lifestyle," Eric says of coping with food allergy. Once he and his wife had made sure that Sebastian's surroundings were safe, carrying around an auto-injector was, he says, "like an afterthought."

DAILY LIFE WITH FOOD ALLERGIES

Living with food allergy means maintaining multiple kinds of vigilance. For parents, there's the ever-present vigilance that never shuts off unless your child is sleeping. There are moments of intense vigilance—at a birthday party, at the playground, at restaurants. And there is the tiny-details vigilance that makes sure relatives, friends, babysitters, and anyone else who may be temporarily caring for your child or providing food for adults with food allergy take the concern as seriously as you do. Life with food allergy often feels like a million small moments of such surveillance, wrapped in worry, with a sparkly bow of feeling like an annoyance stuck on top.

Parents should not hesitate to embrace their inner pesterer. In a 2012 study of more than 500 food-allergic preschool children, under-use of epinephrine was a "substantial problem." We need to be advocates for the food-allergic people in our lives. But also, many parents find they are most comfortable simply bringing their own holiday treats to wherever they're going for celebrations or keeping a small, allergen-free snack always on hand. All those coping with food allergy need to find the approach that suits them best.

Many schools now offer nut-free tables in the cafeteria. These have pros and cons. On the one hand, they hypothetically provide a safe surface for young children unable to supervise themselves. But before parents consign their children to the "allergy table," there are some other considerations. Sitting at a separate table may stigmatize students with food allergy. Such accommodations may also give children a false sense of security, leading them to lower their guard in the very environment where it needs to be up highest.

And parents should also be aware that if a school can't satisfy an allergy-related request, that doesn't make the school an enemy. Jamie Saxena, a nurse practitioner with our team, served the community as a nurse at ten different schools in and around Mountain View, California. She recalls parents asking for the impossible, such as wanting the entire kindergarten class to wash their hands after lunch, a process that would have taken all their recess time. "It's better to help children prepare for reality than give them a false sense of security," says Saxena. We suggest that families consider the full picture and do what's right for the child at the time, but with the flexibility to change as the child grows or as his or her needs change. We also recommend that schools create consensus guidelines that educators across the country can follow, as Canada and Australia have done. Uniform guidelines would ensure that every school's decisions surrounding food allergies are transparent, evidence based, and consistent.

ALTERNATIVE TREATMENTS FOR ALLERGIC REACTIONS

As with all diseases, alternative treatments for food allergy abound. At this time, no rigorous evidence supports interventions beyond avoidance, epinephrine, and the new approaches for preventing and reversing immune-based sensitivity covered in this book.

Herbal formulas rooted in Traditional Chinese Medicine are currently under investigation. In particular, a blend known as food allergy herbal formula-2 (FAHF-2), which includes nine herbs, has been studied in clinical trials. The mix of herbs used in FAHF-2 is based on a classic formula known as Wu Mei Wan, which has been studied for asthma and gastroenteritis. A study in mice showed that FAHF-2 stopped peanut-induced anaphylaxis in mice, and another showed that it also stopped anaphylaxis due to peanut, egg, and fish. After these intriguing results, researchers in New York and Chicago conducted a small clinical trial with 68 people allergic to peanut, tree nut, sesame, fish, shellfish, or any combination of these. The goal of the study was to see if FAHF-2 would stop the immune system from launching an attack against the allergen. The herbal formula proved to be safe, but did not improve the patients' tolerance to their food allergens. It may be that the dose used in the study was inadequate or that the herbs were not taken for long enough. The study authors also noted that many of the participants didn't stick to the prescribed regimen. There may be a role for an altered version of FAHF-2, B-FAHF-2, as an accompaniment to our program for desensitizing the immune system, which we will introduce in a later chapter.

Individuals seeking approaches beyond what Western medicine offers may also come across the work of Xiu-Min Li, a physician in New York City. Dr. Li, an immunologist with extensive training in Traditional Chinese Medicine, has developed herbal formulas intended to ameliorate eczema, food allergy, and asthma. We strongly advise anyone exploring these options to inform their allergist and pediatrician or general practitioner. Some herbs become dangerous in the presence of certain foods or medications, so it is vital to disclose their use, whether as a cream, in a bath, or taken by mouth.

Entering the world of food allergy is like being a stranger in a strange land. The diagnosis raises emotional questions about blame and mistakes that can be especially difficult to deal with in the early months of raising a child. Many parents wonder what they did wrong or what they should have done differently. Adapting to the new reality of food allergy can also be daunting and stressful. Deciphering the confusing language of food labels, speaking with school administrators, even attending a toddler birthday party can cause anxiety that people without food allergy may not understand. And the background hum of worry that becomes the soundtrack of life with food allergy can also leave a family exhausted. In a later chapter, we'll speak extensively about the psychological toll that food allergy can take on families and how to move swiftly through that landscape without becoming stuck. For now, we offer these words: help is available and more is on the way.

THE BOTTOM LINE

- Labeling laws are improving but vary country to country. Those dealing with food allergy should be aware of the regulations in their area.

- Allergic reactions resulting in death from food allergy are extremely rare.

- Anaphylaxis does not refer just to allergic reactions that are life-threatening.

- Epinephrine is a lifesaving medicine that should be used for specific types of allergic reactions. Everyone with food allergies should carry two epinephrine self-injectors.

- "Allergen-free" tables in school cafeterias and classrooms can provide a false sense of security and may be isolating for children suffering from food allergies.

Part II

THE SCIENCE OF TREATING AND REVERSING FOOD ALLERGY

Chapter 5

THE AVOIDANCE MYTH: WHAT WE USED TO THINK

How food allergy became synonymous with fear

It wasn't surprising that a 13-year-old boy with an extreme reaction to eggs ended up on Harley Street in London in the early 1900s. The street had about a hundred doctor's offices and was a known destination for medical care. What was surprising, though, was what happened to the child after he arrived.

The child, whose name is lost to history, had never been able to eat eggs—not meringue, not cake, and definitely not served with bacon, all of which, his parents told Harley Street physician Alfred Schofield, had triggered attacks. The attacks were severe. If he ingested even a minuscule amount of egg, the child began drooling. His lips burned and swelled. He itched. His eyelids grew puffy. Hives covered his body. Normal breathing turned to wheezing as his airway tightened. He once swelled up almost instantly after eating a bun that, although it contained no egg, had been brushed shiny with egg white. His skin blistered when raw egg touched it. His parents told Schofield that their son had had about 150 such attacks in his young life.

Schofield understood that the child's life was at stake. And so in December of 1906, he began a treatment. Schofield made pills, each containing one ten-thousandth of a raw egg, which the child swallowed daily without knowing their contents. A month later, the egg dose was increased to one thousandth. The escalation continued through June, when the portion was raised to one thirty-third. In July, Schofield stopped the pills and gave the child some pudding and cake with egg. By the end of the month, he was consuming an eighth of an egg each day. Then a full egg. Every day. Without any reaction.

Schofield published his case study, "A Case of Egg Poisoning," in *The Lancet* in 1908. He thought the treatment might be unique— he'd never heard of it before—but suspected the publication of it would attract letters from other physicians who knew about the method and had already tried it. According to the scientific literature, no such letters arrived. After a brief blip on the radar of food allergy sufferers, the approach was soon lost for decades. Understanding why requires a brief foray into the history of this perplexing condition.

Food allergy existed long before the egg-allergic child walked into Schofield's clinic. As far back as 2600 BC, Chinese emperors advised pregnant women that eating shrimp, chicken, and meat could give them skin "ulcerations." Hippocrates, who lived from 460 to about 375 BC, noticed that some people had a constitution that was "hostile" to cheese. Around 400 BC, Democritus offered the idea that all matter was made of tiny particles—atoms—that varied in size, shape, and arrangement. If a person couldn't tolerate a certain food, it was because the shape of the atoms in the food didn't fit the shape of the person's gastrointestinal tract. That notion was distilled into poetry around three hundred years later by Titus Lucretius Cato when he wrote, "What is food to one, to another is rank poison."

Galen, the most famous doctor of the Roman empire, noticed that milk and cheese didn't agree with everyone. He thought it might be due to variations in the cows. He wasn't wrong. In the 1900s (AD, that is), researchers discovered that milk from cows that grazed on peanut hay, wheat bran, and ragweed could trigger reactions in people allergic to those plants. A study in 1930 found that breast milk from mothers who ate raw eggs contained egg allergen.

History is littered with revealing clues about our long-running relationship with food allergies. Some ancient Egyptians seemed to believe legumes should be avoided. Some Greco-Roman physicians felt similarly. Moses Maimonides, a twelfth-century rabbi and physician, wrote a "Treatise on Asthma," in which he asserted that milk exacerbated the condition. He also called for avoiding peaches, apricots, and cucumbers. And Richard III, king of England from 1483 to 1485, may have used his strawberry allergy to falsely accuse an adversary of witchcraft.

Scientific literature of centuries past provides another window into our persistent search to understand how to prevent and treat food allergy. Egg allergies in children between the ages of 2 and 16 caused what some doctors described as "alimentary anaphylaxis"— that is, gastrointestinal issues, in addition to hives and asthma. Among nursing infants, milk was the most common trigger. Goat or donkey milk sometimes worked as a substitute, but not always. Wheat appeared problematic for adults. Fish, shellfish, and mollusks gradually entered the fray. A case report from 1656 describes the blister that arose after egg was rubbed onto the skin of an allergic patient. In another, from 1929, a woman's finger turned red where she accidentally pricked it with a needle that had just been used to pierce an eggshell.

The word *allergy* first appeared in 1906, coined by Austrian physician Clemens von Pirquet the same year Alfred Schofield treated the egg-allergic child. (Before then, the disease was referred to as "idiosyncrasy.") He noticed how the skin reacted about a day after a cowpox vaccination. Von Pirquet suspected a link between allergy and the immune system after noticing that children injected with serum from animals sometimes developed a fatal illness that looked an awful lot like the sickness developed by some people as a result of bee stings and certain foods. That wasn't possible, he reasoned, unless the same underlying mechanism drove both reactions. To Von

Pirquet, the word *reaction* didn't seem to cut it as a description for the sequence of events triggered by a vaccine or a food. Neither did *hypersensitivity,* which doctors were using to describe a wide range of phenomena. He wanted a term that applied to the specific phenomenon of the body changing when it encounters some other organic matter, alive or dead. *Allergy,* as Von Pirquet defined it, simply meant "a deviation from the original state or normal behavior of the individual." (The word comes from the Greek *allos,* meaning "other," and *ergon*, meaning "work".) His definition was a bit too broad, but it helped turn the eyes of food allergy researchers toward immune malfunction as a cause.

Von Pirquet had one more major contribution to make to the world of food allergy. In 1907, he started scratching people's skin with a bit of tuberculin bacteria as a way to test people for tuberculosis, a highly contagious disease. If the test came out positive, then Von Pirquet knew the individual was infected with the bacteria. Other responses, depending on the age of the individual and whether they'd had tuberculosis or other infectious diseases, delivered other crucial information. It was the first skin prick test, a hallmark of allergy care. In 1912, a pediatrician named Oscar Schloss showed that Von Pirquet's method could be used to test children for allergies to egg, almond, and oat. Soon after, a group of doctors confirmed the effectiveness of skin prick tests for food allergy after rubbing buckwheat into the skin of a patient who'd suffered hives, swelling, and other symptoms after consuming it (before this patient, buckwheat poisoning had been seen only in cows).

A food allergy diagnosis often begins with a skin prick test. Of course in this situation it's not tuberculosis bacteria but food that is in question. This widely known test entails pricking a person's skin to allow a drop of solution containing a suspected food allergen to seep into the body. The test is usually done on the forearm or back and often includes multiple foods at once. The idea is that the solution contains enough of a protein to trigger a response by the immune system. If a person is allergic to a certain food, their skin will show it with a wheal—a raised bump surrounded by itchy, red skin—within about half an hour. (We'll delve further into diagnosing food allergy below.)

Skin prick testing became a popular method for diagnosing food allergy in the early twentieth century, in part because it was the only tool allergists had for doing so. And after an allergy was diagnosed, many clinicians turned to desensitization for treatment. They injected minute amounts of allergen extracts into their patients' bodies, slowly increasing the amount incrementally until, like Schofield's patient, the immune system became desensitized. The protein that was once an enemy had become a harmless friend.

But all was not resolved for people living with food allergy. Skin prick testing suffered from a major problem, one that continues to plague it today: false positives. An estimated 50 percent or more of skin prick tests deliver bad results, indicating that people are allergic to a particular food when they aren't. Sometimes the tool used for the test was faulty. At other times, the skill and experience of the tester was lacking. Or the extract placed in the skin was poor quality. Sometimes the opposite occurred and the test missed a potentially dangerous food allergy (false negatives are extremely rare with skin prick tests these days).

As problems with skin prick tests emerged, some clinicians started to wonder if food allergy worked differently than, say, allergies to pollen or bee stings. They theorized that because skin prick tests got food allergy wrong so often, the inner workings of the disease must be different from that of other allergies. The tests failed, they figured, because the immune system didn't react to foods the same way it did to those other allergens. That suspicion turned out to be completely wrong. But at the time, this logic led clinicians to conclude that desensitization probably wouldn't work, either. These doctors began referring to themselves as "food allergists," thus carving out a distinct field within the world of allergy care.

They weren't wrong to doubt the effectiveness of desensitization. In 1921, a 1-year-old baby nearly died—twice—from a skin test for egg allergy. Desensitization treatments also led to several deaths in the following years. Clearly, the food allergists of the day came to believe, this was not the appropriate way to treat food allergy.

Enter the elimination diet, introduced in the 1920s as an alternative method for diagnosing food allergy and step toward treatment. The concept is credited to an allergist from California named Albert Rowe, who first wrote about the method in 1926 and published a book on it in 1941. The elimination diet is exactly what it sounds like: All potential allergens are omitted from what a person eats. They are introduced back into the diet one by one, with waits of days between adding the next food back in. The approach enables a person to isolate the culprit allergen; if the immune system reacts to a given food upon reintroduction, then clearly that's the culprit allergen. But the diets could be grueling. Rowe crafted intensive meal plans for patients to follow. And because he was checking a wide range of possible allergens, each of which required at least a couple of days for reintroduction, diagnosing a food allergy through an elimination diet could take years. A patient undertaking an elimination diet, Rowe wrote, had to be "intelligent and understanding." Once the slow reintroduction of foods pinpointed the culprit allergen, the prescription was simple: avoidance. Eliminate the bad food permanently. This, allergists came to believe, was the best, if not only, treatment. Keep away from the food at all costs.

Matters were growing tense by the early 1930s. Using elimination tests to diagnose food allergy rankled traditional allergists. Even though they knew that skin prick tests could be faulty, they still considered them the gold standard. If a food allergy couldn't be detected with a skin prick, then it probably didn't exist, they said. The fact that elimination diets depended so much on patient participation irritated these doctors, who believed this dynamic made for shaky conclusions. This position grew more extreme in the years to come. By the 1950s, some allergists voiced the notion that food allergy could sometimes be psychosomatic, a figment of the imagination. Sometimes, they said, a session on a psychiatrist's couch would be the best treatment. Right around this time, a few well-known food allergists took just the opposite position. Not only was food allergy real but it was possibly responsible for many more health complaints than physicians had realized. For a time, food allergy became a catchall way to explain everything that medicine couldn't.

Thus a division was born. In the 1960s, the broader field of allergy specialists began shunning food allergy as a legitimate medical specialty. Physicians who'd once been interested in pursuing treatments for the condition turned their attention toward other fields that their colleagues accepted and approved. Those who remained dedicated to food allergy as their specific focus were left with little support to advance the research. That split, along with the dismissal of food allergy research as a worthy and important pursuit, stymied progress.

Then came the uptick in peanut allergy. Fatalities began piling into medical literature in the late 1980s. A 1989 report on seven worldwide deaths due to peanut allergy warned that this condition was "probably the most common cause of death by food anaphylaxis in the United States." In 1990, the *British Medical Journal* published pages of letters emphasizing the dangers of peanut allergy. "Peanut allergy is the most worrisome food allergy issue confronting the pediatrician today," stated one 1992 report. "Of all the potentially allergenic foods, peanut appears to be the most dangerous." Rising rates of peanut allergy and fatal reactions began making news headlines. "Peanut Allergies Have Put Sufferers on Constant Alert," ran one *Wall Street Journal* headline in 1995. A 1999 report estimated that 1.1 percent of the U.S. population (3 million people) was allergic to peanuts.

But as food allergy rates rose, the medical establishment had little to offer aside from the same advice from decades earlier: avoid the allergen at all costs. The rift among physicians interested in food allergy had left the field frozen in time. In 1976, an influential paper on food allergy in the medical journal *American Family Physician* pronounced: "Treatment is avoidance. Desensitization does not work." Food allergy care was exactly where it was when Rowe popularized elimination diets as a diagnosis in the 1930s. Forty years later, most medical professionals had nothing else to say on the matter.

THE PREVENTION DIET

Just as avoidance appeared to be the best way to treat allergy, it also seemed like the best way to prevent it. Back in 1934, two pediatricians from Chicago looked at rates of eczema among babies who were exclusively breastfed, those who were breastfed and also had milk-based formula, and those who had only formula. They reported that seven times as many babies in the formula-only group had eczema compared to the breast-milk-only group. A handful of similar studies followed in the 1980s and 1990s. In the mid-1980s, a study in mice found that delaying the introduction of food proteins known to trigger allergic reactions averted the development of antibodies to those proteins. More importantly, studies in people showed the same effect. In 1989, a group from California reported the results of their randomized study investigating avoidance as a tactic for preventing food allergy. A group of 103 mothers avoided milk, egg, and peanut during the last three months of their pregnancy and while breastfeeding. Their babies did not eat solid foods until they were 6 months old. They had no milk, corn, soy, citrus, or wheat until they were a year old, and no peanut, egg, or fish until they were 2 years old. The other group, which included 185 mothers, had no limits on their diets and followed the recommended guidelines at the time for feeding their babies. The authors reported that the avoidance group had significantly lower rates of allergy. Interestingly, they noted that the group that had avoided potential allergens had just slightly lower levels of IgE, a hallmark of allergy (the presence of IgE antibodies doesn't always indicate an allergy, but there are no food allergies without IgE antibodies). Still, the researchers concluded that avoiding allergenic foods "reduced food sensitization and allergy during the first year of life." Another study that same year found that infants who had no milk during their first six months and whose mothers avoided eggs, milk, and fish during the first three months of breastfeeding had less eczema during that time period than infants whose mothers followed an unrestricted diet. The difference disappeared after 6 months of age. In 2003, a German study of 945 infants concluded that keeping babies away from milk during the first year of life prevented an allergy to it. "Prevention of allergic diseases in the first year of life is feasible by means of dietary intervention," the authors noted. By "intervention," of course, they meant avoidance.

And so the avoidance paradigm took hold. The best way to prevent food allergy in children, the experts said, was to keep potential threats out of the diet for the first months of life. Some foods, like peanuts, were best avoided for the first two years. Official recommendations advising parents to delay the introduction of common allergens into their children's diets poured in. Beginning in 1998, UK health authorities suggested when peanut allergy ran in the family, children should avoid this food until they turned 3 years old. The American Academy of Pediatrics (AAP) followed suit starting in 2000, advising that children should hold off on dairy until 1 year of age, eggs until 2 years, and peanuts, tree nuts, and fish until 3 years.

In 2003, the AAP and two pediatric medical societies in Europe published guidelines reiterating the belief that introducing commonly problematic foods too early increased the risk of food allergy in children. The agencies had some differences. The AAP recommended that pregnant women consider avoiding peanuts and that nursing mothers eliminate peanuts and consider also eliminating eggs, milk, and fish. The two European organizations (the European Society for Paediatric Allergology and Clinical Immunology and the European Society for Paediatric Gastroenterology, Hepatology and Nutrition) did not suggest that approach. However, they did note that because peanuts aren't essential to the diet, pregnant women might as well avoid them.

As for the babies, all three agencies suggested avoiding soy formula. The two European organizations suggested starting solid foods at the fifth month of life, with no particular restrictions due to a lack of data. By 2008, however, most pediatric authorities in most countries recommended holding off on milk until a baby reached its first birthday. Allergists at Mount Sinai and Duke University voiced concern about the growing practice of delayed introduction. The European Society for Paediatric Gastroenterology, Hepatology and Nutrition did, too. But the forces of caution and fear were too strong to stop.

And so it was that the notion of omitting potential allergens from a baby's diet took hold. Pregnant women stopped eating peanuts and dairy. New parents often delayed the introduction of solid foods until their babies were 6 months old. One inquiry found that 20 percent of German mothers were postponing the introduction of solid foods until after 6 months. Peanuts became the enemy of early toddlerhood. There was only one way to prevent food allergy, the thinking went, and that was to treat the food as an enemy before it even entered the body. But basing recommendations on small or weak studies can go very wrong.

THE PROBLEM WITH AVOIDANCE

As the dogma of avoidance took hold, so did something else: a rise in food allergy rates. Wherever pediatric authorities recommended holding off on peanuts, eggs, and the like until 1 or 2 or 3 years of age, the prevalence in allergy to those exact foods spiked, researchers in the UK reported in 2016. Even if avoidance wasn't responsible for the dramatic rise in food allergy, one fact was clear: avoidance also wasn't making the problem go away. If delaying the introduction of certain foods could prevent allergy, then why were rates not declining among children? With such a short span of time between birth and the onset of allergy, we didn't need to wait long to see the change that avoidance promised to bring—yet it never came.

The persistence of food allergy under the reign of avoidance prompted some physicians to scrutinize the data. What did the scientific research really show about avoidance? A large group of researchers from across Europe decided to take a look. They scoured the medical literature for studies focused on preventing sensitization and/or full-blown food allergy. They kept their criteria strict, not considering studies examining the incidence of symptoms, only those with actual diagnoses as part of their data. A total of seventy-four studies fit their requirements. A close look at them dismantled the avoidance paradigm.

This study of studies found no evidence that avoiding potential allergens during pregnancy helped prevent the condition in babies. "There is no strong evidence to recommend changes to the diet of pregnant women to prevent food allergy in infants," the authors wrote. The same was true for the diet during breastfeeding. Some evidence showed a benefit for exclusive breastfeeding over combining nursing with formula, but other evidence showed that "extended exclusive breastfeeding" could also increase the risk of food allergy. As for delaying the introduction of solid foods, the data spoke clearly. The practice showed no benefit in protecting high-risk children against food allergy, the researchers found. For children with a normal risk of food allergy, delaying the introduction of solid foods until after four months didn't reduce the likelihood of food allergy. In fact, two of the studies they looked at showed that introducing foods before four months might actually lower the risk. Another showed that infants who ate fish were less likely to develop a fish allergy. Delaying milk also accomplished nothing for parents wishing to prevent food allergy in their babies. In short, the evidence behind avoidance was scarce, and the data that existed did not make a strong case for the practice. Rather, it was just the opposite. "Changes to infant diet such as delaying the introduction of solid foods," the authors wrote, "are unlikely to protect against food allergy."

The authors did note that dietary modifications might be helpful only if this approach is combined with certain changes to the child's environment. The SPACE (Study on the Prevention of Allergy in Children in Europe) trial had reported that protective measures against exposure to dust-mite allergens could be protective against both airborne and food allergy. And a 2007 study of 120 infants on the Isle of Wight showed the same thing for infants who were at high risk of food allergy because it ran in their families. A handful of other studies in the seventy-four-study review showed a similar trend: for children with a family predisposition to food allergy, some dietary alterations in the earliest months of life (mainly, some restrictions on nursing mothers and avoiding milk formula) were tied to a lower risk of food allergy, but mostly only when families also reduced the infant's exposure to dust mites and tobacco smoke. These are important findings, but they apply only to the first few months of life for infants in families already predisposed to food allergy. The bulk of the evidence shows that delaying the introduction of common allergens such as egg, milk, and peanut does not reduce the likelihood of developing food allergy. In fact, evidence accruing during the first decade of the twenty-first century showed that delayed introduction could actually be increasing that likelihood.

In 2010, the National Institute of Allergy and Infectious Diseases (NIAID), part of the National Institutes of Health, convened an expert panel to establish guidelines for diagnosing and managing food allergy. By this point, the peanut-paranoid writing was on the wall. The panel combed through the evidence yet again and found it wanting where delayed introduction was concerned. There was enough data to recommend exclusive breastfeeding until 4 to 6 months of age if possible. But they did not recommend altering the mother's diet during pregnancy or while nursing. They did not recommend the use of soy formula instead of milk formula to reduce the risk of food allergy, although they did find evidence favoring hydrolyzed formula for infants who are at risk of food allergy and not breastfed exclusively. And when it came to considering when parents should introduce potential food allergens to their babies, the panel saw no reason to recommend delays. "Insufficient evidence exists for delaying introduction of solid foods, including potentially allergenic foods, beyond 4 to 6 months of age," the guidelines stated, "even in infants at risk of developing allergic disease." The earlier recommendation by the American Academy of Pediatrics and other medical authorities to delay the introduction of common allergens was officially outdated. In 2012, a committee with the American Academy of Allergy, Asthma, and Immunology advised beginning a diverse diet of solid foods beginning at 4 to 6 months of age.

Incidentally, the NIAID panel also looked at whether the presence of environmental allergens truly exacerbated the risk of food allergy. They found no evidence that avoiding dust mites, pollen, or pet dander had any effect on food allergy whatsoever. (As we will discuss later, having a pet may actually reduce the risk of food allergy.)

A Timeline of Food Allergy Diagnosis and Treatment

~75 BC: Roman philosopher Titus Lucretius Cato states, "What is food to one, to another is rank poison," in his poem *De Rerum Natura.*

~1180: Moses Maimonides advises asthmatic Prince Al-Afdal, son of King Saladin, to avoid milk, nuts, and legumes.

1865: Charles H. Blackley develops the scratch test for allergy to grass pollen, the first modern diagnostic test for allergy.

1906: Clemens von Pirquet coins the term *allergy.*

1908: British physician Alfred Schofield treats a case of egg allergy by feeding the patient small amounts of egg.

1912: The first scratch test for food allergy (egg) becomes available.

1920s: Physicians begin using the skin prick test to diagnose allergy.

1926: Albert Rowe introduces his elimination diet method as a food allergy treatment.

1942: First antihistamine used medicinally.

1950: Discovery of mast cells, which are involved in food allergy.

1966: Two labs simultaneously discover IgE, the immune cells that drive food allergy reactions.

1973: The first blood test for food allergy becomes available.

1987: The FDA approves the first modern epinephrine auto-injector, the EpiPen.

1997: The first study of subcutaneous (injection) immunotherapy for peanut allergy.

2003: Sublingual immunotherapy proves safe for people allergic to kiwi.

2010: Epicutaneous immunotherapy proves safe for children allergic to milk.

2010: National Institute of Allergy and Infectious Diseases expert panel says that delayed introduction does not prevent food allergies.

2011: Oral immunotherapy plus omalizumab effectively treats milk allergy.

2014: Oral immunotherapy plus omalizumab effectively treats multiple allergies simultaneously.

2019: A phase 3 study of the "peanut patch" successfully desensitizes patients to peanuts.

2019: A phase 3 study of AR101 (peanut flour) successfully desensitizes patients to peanuts.

2019: An FDA advisory committee approves AR101, leading to the first FDA approval for a food allergy treatment.

WHY AVOIDANCE DOESN'T WORK

The idea that delaying the introduction of risky foods would prevent allergy was somewhat understandable. Infant immune systems are vulnerable. Waiting until they become stronger could help avoid violent reactions to what are actually harmless substances. But in reality, acquainting the immune system with innocuous foreign matter—peanuts, eggs, fish—early in life allows it to become familiar with these foods at the same time it is getting to know other frequently encountered substances.

The proponents of delayed introduction had also neglected to take into account environmental exposure to common allergens. If you eat peanuts in your house, researchers from the UK and Portugal reported in 2013, then peanut protein will get into your household dust. Peanut residue lingers for three hours on hands and in saliva. If children have eczema, then they are especially prone to exposure through their skin. As we discussed in chapter 2, when the immune system is exposed to certain proteins through the skin first, instead of by mouth, then it may be more likely to treat those proteins as an enemy. By not feeding them to a child, we fail to teach the child's immune system soon enough that these proteins are actually foods. Peanut dust entering the bloodstream through the rough skin on a patch of eczema should ideally not be an immune system's initial meet and greet with this protein. It's understandable that the immune system would develop an antagonistic response to a protein that shouldn't be entering our bodies through our skin. But if the immune system already recognizes that protein as a food, then it's less likely to treat it as harmful when it comes through the skin.

As we'll see in the next chapter, introducing foods early isn't just safe. It's a tool for prevention.

TESTING, TESTING

Nikki Godwin had a hard time figuring out what her daughter, Sabrina, was allergic to. The problem began with eczema, which appeared when Sabrina was just 10 weeks old and worsened over time. Her pediatrician thought she might have a dairy allergy and suggested that Nikki, who was breastfeeding, stay away from milk. But then Sabrina developed hives while she was nursing. Nikki brought Sabrina to an allergist, where she tested positive for egg allergy. "I thought I had learned what she was allergic to at that point," says Nikki.

But months later, a giant welt arose on Sabrina's cheek where Nikki kissed her after eating a peanut butter and jelly sandwich. Nikki wondered if her daughter could be allergic to peanuts, but for some reason the thought seemed silly. She already knew what Sabrina was allergic to—egg. The allergist had advised her to delay the introduction of peanuts because one allergy often indicates others. But the idea that her daughter had multiple food allergies seemed farfetched. Then one day when Sabrina was a year old, her grandmother gave her a big spoonful of peanut butter. Within minutes she was covered in hives, itchy and restless. Soon a strange cough began. They bundled Sabrina up for an emergency trip to the pediatrician. They returned to the allergist for more testing. Sabrina, it turned out, was allergic to peanuts and also tree nuts.

The allergist told Nikki that her daughter should also avoid sesame seeds. Nikki had never heard of a child being allergic to egg, peanuts, and tree nuts. Surely she couldn't also be allergic to sesame. At a restaurant with few options for her young and allergic daughter, Nikki ordered Sabrina some hummus, which contains sesame seed paste. "The first bite was probably her fastest and worst allergic reaction yet," Nikki recalls. A test confirmed what the hives had revealed. Sabrina was indeed allergic to sesame.

When her younger daughter, Simone, was born, Nikki couldn't imagine that she would be allergic, too. Then one day Simone broke out in hives after eating half of a chewy Spree candy. A year or so later, she had the same reaction to the same candy. Nikki looked up the ingredients and found out the candy was made with egg. Simone, an allergy test later confirmed, had all the same allergies as her big sister.

Because food allergy can have a dramatic impact on one's life, making sure of the diagnosis is crucial. A single reaction doesn't always indicate a chronic allergy. Not all symptoms are driven by the presence of IgE antibodies geared to attack a food protein. Sometimes testing ferrets out additional allergies after a reaction to a food; Nikki's daughters tested positive for allergies to tree nuts even though they had never eaten them. Or sometimes an immune system harbors those antibodies, but the person can tolerate the food perfectly fine. In other words, food allergy isn't always cut-and-dried, so it's best to confirm the condition with a test.

And yet testing doesn't always provide a clear answer. Although many people are familiar with the skin prick test, for example, this method is fallible, frequently delivering false positives. In this chapter, we will cover all that you need to know in order to feel assured that a diagnosis—whether it confirms or refutes the presence of an allergy—is accurate and reliable.

MEDICAL HISTORY

The first step for those who suspect they have a food allergy is providing their medical history to a pediatrician, general practitioner, or allergist. For children, parents must be able to relay accurate details of allergic reactions, along with any family history of such problems.

The world of food allergy has been somewhat tainted by a history of exaggerated claims. In the past, complaints of food-triggered reactions haven't been confirmed by rigorous allergy tests. More recently, sociologists have raised concerns that hype surrounding peanut allergy has made us more fearful than we should be, even going so far as to conclude that there is no epidemic. And we humans are very subject to bias, faulty recollections, and other weaknesses that could lead us to believe we have a food allergy when we don't.

All of these factors crop up in food allergy, as they do in many areas of medicine. We are fallible, sometimes easily swayed, and not as reliable as we'd like to think we are. However, these lapses have led some health professionals to view food allergy concerns with understandable skepticism—and sometimes a dangerous level of dismissal. That's why it's crucial for parents of potentially allergic children or adults experiencing symptoms for the first time to provide accurate details. Information you will want to provide to your doctors includes:

- When did the reaction happen?
- What were the symptoms?
- What foods had the patient eaten?
- What foods were nearby?
- How many times did the reaction occur?
- How long did it take to see the symptoms?
- How long did it take for symptoms to resolve on each occasion?
- How did you treat the symptoms?
- Do any other members of your family have food allergies?
- Do you (or your child) have dry skin, eczema, or asthma?

Of course providing these details isn't always feasible. When your child is breaking out in hives and starting to wheeze, you're probably not stopping to write down all the foods she may have touched. That would be difficult since most first reactions occur from foods that contain one or more allergens—a granola bar, a cookie, soup—rather than the single allergen itself. That's fine. An allergist can try to diagnose food allergy without this information. If you are on the receiving end of too much doubt, it may be time to seek a second opinion. But the more information you can offer, the better.

Medical histories are also essential because the symptoms may be caused by another problem entirely. Plenty of other medical conditions can lead us to react badly to certain foods. But before you go scaring yourself with Dr. Google, rest assured that it is possible to detect the condition conclusively. If you suspect a food allergy, see a doctor and leave the web searching for another day.

FOOD DIARIES

Keeping a food diary can be helpful for the diagnosis. Writing down meals avoids the pitfalls of memory. And the list of items may help a doctor dig out a hidden culprit. Soy protein could have been added to a prepared food. Fruit juice may have been packaged on a factory line that handles milk as well. A reaction to pasta may be due to an allergy to egg rather than to wheat. Allergists know the trends to look for. A patient once came to our clinic after suffering reactions to oatmeal cookies, pumpkin pie, and chai tea. A careful analysis of her diet revealed cinnamon as a possible culprit because it was in each of the foods. Subsequent testing confirmed that suspicion was correct. Children tend to be most susceptible to the most common allergens, whereas adults often develop allergies we're not as accustomed to. A diary can reveal a source of contamination—a problematic food crossing paths with a harmless food, unbeknownst to us—and it may provide surprising information about an undetected underlying health issue.

SKIN PRICK TEST

The skin prick test is the diagnostic we most commonly associate with food allergy. We recommend that children or adults who show signs of food allergy be checked with this method, which tests for the presence of IgE antibodies to suspected allergens. With this test, a medical professional uses a simple device to lightly puncture the skin on the forearm or the back, and then inserts extracts from suspected allergens where the skin has been broken. The allergy shows itself within thirty minutes; a wheal—a raised white bump surrounded by reddened skin—indicates its presence. A wheal greater than about 3 millimeters, or greater than the skin's reaction to a control (a puncture without a food extract inserted), is considered positive.

Skin prick tests pose very little risk, even for people with severe allergy. However, anyone seeking this test to diagnose a food allergy should be aware of the high rate of false positives. Skin prick tests are less than 50 percent accurate than the most rigorous diagnostic (discussed below). Many people will react to the allergen extract even though they don't have an actual allergy. As a result, people may believe themselves allergic to a certain food when that food is perfectly safe. That scenario can be particularly precarious for a baby or toddler, for if a family avoids giving a false-positive allergen to a child, then the food could end up becoming an allergen as a result of the delayed introduction.

False negatives are extremely rare—a no-allergy result is correct 95 percent of the time—and so these tests are effective for ruling out food allergy. However, babies under 2 years of age are particularly prone to having smaller wheals, which an allergist may mistakenly interpret as a negative result. Skin that has been treated for eczema may also produce smaller wheals because the steroid creams used to treat this condition can dampen allergic reactions. And the extracts inserted into pricked skin, which are usually prepared commercially, may not have the proteins that trigger allergies to certain fruits and vegetables, such as apples, oranges, and carrots.

Think of it this way: If your skin prick test is positive—the wheal is at least 3 millimeters larger than the inert control—then you *might* have a food allergy. If your test is negative—the wheal is smaller than the control or nonexistent—then you almost certainly do not have a food allergy. Another chief benefit of a skin prick test is that it narrows down the culprit allergen when patients or doctors suspect several candidates.

BLOOD TEST

Like a skin prick test, a blood test also hunts for IgE antibodies. Also like skin prick tests, blood tests suffer from a false-positive rate of 50 percent or more. Blood tests can be costly. Also, the results may be misleading—a person may test positive for an allergy to a protein that is related to an allergen, but that does not in and of itself pose a threat. For example, a person with peanut allergy may test positive for a grass pollen allergy only because the two proteins are similar.

Blood tests aren't recommended as a tried and true method for confirming a food allergy. Some allergists may offer these tests to corroborate the results of a skin prick test. But because both approaches have a high likelihood of delivering incorrect information, that combination may not deliver more reliable reading than either test alone.

DIAGNOSTIC TESTS FOR FOOD ALLERGIES				
TEST	HOW OFTEN DOES THIS TEST PROVIDE FALSE-NEGATIVE RESULTS?	HOW OFTEN DOES THIS TEST PROVIDE FALSE-POSITIVE RESULTS?	IS THIS TEST USEFUL FOR DIAGNOSING FOOD ALLERGY?	IS THIS TEST MADE BY A LICENSED LABORATORY, APPROVED FOR PHYSICIAN USE, AND COVERED BY INSURANCE?
IgE-ImmunoCAP	Infrequently	Frequently	Sometimes	Yes
IgE to components	Infrequently	Frequently	Sometimes	Yes
IgG	Unknown	Unknown	No	No
Basophil activation test	Infrequently	Infrequently	Sometimes	No, it's still experimental
Skin prick test	Very infrequently	Frequently	Sometimes	Yes
Skin patch test	Frequently	Frequently	No	No
Intradermal test	Infrequently	Very frequently	No	No

INTRADERMAL, PATCH, AND OTHER TESTS

Several other tests purport to effectively diagnose food allergy. We recommend avoiding these unproven tests, which may deliver dubious readings on your food allergy status. IgG/IgG4 testing scans the blood for these antibodies, which contribute to the fight against allergenic foods. However, IgG and IgG4 show up whenever the body fights infections and sometimes as a normal response to benign foods. A test that checks strands of hair for mineral content is based on the flawed rationale that protein remnants of an allergen should show up there (hair grows too slowly for this approach to work). With an intradermal test, sometimes used after a negative skin prick test result, the allergen is injected right into the skin. These tests have a high false-positive rate. Patch tests entail taping the allergen to the back for forty-eight hours and then checking the skin three to four days later for a reaction, an approach that delivers unreliable results and has little evidence supporting its use.

ORAL FOOD CHALLENGE—THE GOLD STANDARD

The only absolutely conclusive test for food allergy is the oral food challenge. With a food challenge, the patient consumes small doses of a suspected allergen. After each dose, the allergist watches for reactions. If none arise, then the dose is increased a little bit. Eventually the dose is high enough to trigger even the mildest food allergy. If no reaction occurs, then no allergy exists. The process usually takes a few hours and must be done by a medical professional. Oral food challenges are designed to provoke a reaction, so it's vital that the equipment to treat allergy symptoms is on hand and ready for immediate use. If an oral food challenge triggers a reaction, the reaction is treated right away.

Even better—the best test of all, really—is the double-blind, placebo-controlled food challenge, or DBPCFC. Verified in the early 1980s as the gold standard for diagnosing food allergy by Colorado-based pediatricians Charles May and S. Allan Bock, it has never been surpassed by any other method since. With this rigorous approach, a patient receives both a suspected allergen and a placebo, given at different times separated by hours or sometimes days. These substances may be given in food, such as pudding or applesauce. Neither the patient nor the doctor knows which item is the allergen and which is the placebo. One test may use peanut powder mixed into applesauce or chocolate pudding, and the next one may test an inert powder mixed into these familiar foods.

The DBPCFC is effective because it eliminates bias. A person worried about a milk allergy may be more prone to feeling symptoms after drinking milk even when the allergy is nonexistent. Similarly, a doctor who is skeptical of a patient's claim or unaware of that person's hypochondria has no grounds to doubt one test more than the other in the double-blind challenge. When multiple food allergies are at play, the DBPCFC isolates which food causes which symptoms.

In another variation on this theme, the food challenge may be single-blinded, which means the doctor knows which test contains the allergen and which contains the placebo, but the patient does not. Again, this approach helps eliminate anything that could influence the outcome aside from an actual allergic reaction. Some clinics opt for an open food challenge, in which everyone knows what's what. This approach works well for people who do not feel anxious about having an allergy.

All these challenges are done in one visit over several hours. The test begins with a tiny dose of the suspected allergen. The exact amount depends on the allergen. Pistachio challenges start with just 1 milligram of the nut, for example. Peanut challenges may start with the equivalent of a tenth of a nut, provided in the form of peanut flour. After enough time passes to be sure that no reaction is imminent, then the dose is increased a bit. Then a bit more and a bit more until it's high enough to be absolutely certain that the patient is not allergic. The ability to consume a full egg white, for example, assures us that the patient is not allergic to egg. For milk, the threshold is about four ounces. Parents prepare to spend most of their day at the clinic, with books and toys for their children. An oral food challenge can be an intense experience for families, but it's worth it for the conclusive answer it provides about a suspected allergy.

There are occasions when an oral food challenge isn't recommended—namely, if a person has already suffered from life-threatening anaphylaxis. In this case, the danger of consuming the food does not outweigh the benefit of confirming the allergy. The trip to the emergency room and documented medical records are often all the confirmation we need. And, of course, if a person is eating the food in their diet without reactions, a food challenge is unnecessary.

BASOPHIL ACTIVATION TEST

Skin prick tests and blood tests lack reliability. Oral food challenges are reliable but time consuming and essentially force the patient into an allergic reaction. Given these options, it's understandable that researchers have been working to develop another. This is where the basophil activation test comes in.

Basophils are white blood cells produced in the bone marrow and circulating in our blood. Like mast cells, basophils have landing strips for IgE antibodies and become activated when these antibodies arrive on site in response to an enemy food protein. Often within just seconds, activated basophils start releasing histamines and other chemicals that trigger all the symptoms we recognize as an allergy attack. Their role has spurred the creation of a test that measures basophils specifically.

The first basophil activation tests (BATs) emerged a few years ago. The tests measure the extent to which the basophils in a sample of blood have become activated after encountering a candidate allergen. The approach has proven effective for diagnosing several food allergies (along with allergies to pollen, latex, venom, and some medications). Studies suggest that it can be used as an additional test to confirm wheat allergy or as part of diagnosing a milk allergy. It may help distinguish food allergy from food sensitivity. It can also be used to test whether a person is likely to be allergic to a particular food.

But the test hasn't been widely adopted because it has some problems. Preserving the cells at the right temperature and testing them while they're still viable has proven tricky. Also, the tests aren't standardized, which means two allergists may come to different conclusions about the same patient.

At Stanford University, a research team that includes mechanical engineers, biophysicists, and basophil experts Steve Galli, Sindy Tang, and Mindy Tsai is developing a microfluidic BAT. The test offers a uniformity that has been absent from the efforts thus far, which makes it more versatile and opens the door for a more standardized approach. The Stanford team is also taking the test several steps further in terms of practicality by creating a device that uses smartphones to match the blood sample with its food nemesis. Although the device is still in development, it could be revolutionary where food allergy testing is concerned. A blood sample is injected into a small device that then plugs into a smartphone jack. An app "reads" the basophil activation levels for peanut, milk, egg, tree nut, and other frequent culprits. The program then prompts users to record their diet and anything they were exposed to in their environment that could exacerbate a food allergy. The data from everyone using this test is also brought together to help researchers identify the causes of food allergy. And the test is fast and inexpensive.

The main message we have regarding food allergy testing is *get tested*. Reactions can be unpredictable; mild symptoms on one occasion don't mean mild symptoms next time. Individuals who suspect they may have a food allergy have nothing to lose from being tested— and everything to gain.

THE BOTTOM LINE

- If you have an adverse reaction to a food, seek testing for food allergies at a clinic with a board-certified allergist and immunology specialist.

- Keep a food diary to assist the physician in making a diagnosis.

- The skin prick test is the most common method for diagnosing food allergy. Blood tests measure the level of IgE antibodies against a food protein. The basophil activation test is more recent and mainly used in research because its use is not yet standardized. No other medical test is appropriate for diagnosing food allergy.

- The oral food challenge is the gold standard for diagnosing a food allergy. This approach separates true food allergy from food sensitization. These tests typically trigger allergic reactions.

Chapter 6

TURNING THE TABLES: THE SCIENCE — AND HOW-TOS — OF EARLY INTRODUCTION

How debunking the avoidance myth transformed medical recommendations

A MYSTERIOUS DIFFERENCE

Gideon Lack was puzzled. A pediatric allergist at King's College London, Lack had watched the alarming rise of peanut allergy in the late 1990s and early 2000s. He had watched rates double in just ten years. And he had seen the disturbing data showing that avoiding food allergens during pregnancy, nursing, and infancy—the very measure health authorities had recommended to stop the problem— had failed.

Questions about the human immune system had first gripped ·him years earlier. Lack was training at Albert Einstein College of Medicine, in New York City, during the AIDS epidemic of the 1980s. But it was his next exposure to immunity that gave him his first clue about food allergy. As part of a group in Denver, Colorado, Lack was trying to treat mice for asthma that had been caused by exposure to egg. The first step was to make the mice allergic to egg, which he tried to do by feeding them bits of the food. His method didn't work. It turned out that science had already figured out that mice would not become allergic to something they'd already eaten. "They develop tolerance by eating," said Lack. Then he realized another researcher in his group was inducing the allergy by exposing patches of slightly irritated skin on the mice to ovalbumin, the main protein in egg white. That approach worked. But at the time, Lack made no connection from this to human allergy.

Back in London in the 1990s, new mothers were asking Lack how their babies could possibly be allergic to peanuts when they'd avoided them entirely during pregnancy. "It became very clear to me that avoidance wasn't working." But he didn't know why.

In the early 1990s, he came across a curious study from the Netherlands on nickel allergy. He knew that people who wear jewelry made with nickel or other metals sometimes develop a rash underneath. The study found that people with pierced ears were less likely to be allergic to nickel if they'd worn orthodontic braces before having their ears pierced. A 1996 study by researchers in Norway and Finland found the same association: braces before ear piercing meant lower rates of nickel allergy. Nickel exposure through the mouth, it seemed, protected people against the allergy they might have had through skin exposure. "In other words," says Lack, "the story of mice could be applicable to humans." But he didn't know why.

He had a couple of possible explanations. Children who weren't eating risky foods were still developing allergies. So maybe it wasn't eating the foods that posed the risk, Lack reasoned. Maybe they were exposed to the food in some other way and that alternate route was triggering the sensitivity. He also wondered if tolerance depended on early exposure by mouth to certain foods. Maybe that was just how the body worked.

Then came a serendipitous trip to Israel. The Israel Association of Allergy and Clinical Immunology had asked him to give a talk in Tel Aviv about peanut allergy. As was his custom when giving such talks, he asked for a show of hands for how many people had seen a case of peanut allergy in the last year. In the UK, he knew, the room would have been full of raised hands. But in Israel, just two or three of the clinicians in the audience put their hands up.

During that trip, he went out to lunch with some friends; he tried the snack that a mother in his group was giving to her baby. He was shocked to discover it tasted like peanut butter. The friends told him that virtually all babies in Israel eat this particular snack.

Lack knew the evidence revealing that infants with severe eczema are at greater risk for allergy. Lotions to treat eczema that contained peanut oil also increased the risk. One study had found that infants with peanut allergy were exposed to peanuts through their environment—oil or peanut dust left on the hands, a kiss on the cheek from lips carrying remnants of a PB&J—ten times more often than infants without peanut allergy. The idea that even when babies didn't consume peanuts by mouth they were still encountering the allergenic protein found further grounding in the fact, as Helen Brough and her team in London found, that this protein remains on the hands and in the saliva in high quantities after the meal or snack is over. Bits of egg, milk, and fish have even been found floating around in house dust. Could it be that ingesting a food early in life was key to tolerating it? In some investigations, just a single dose was enough to make the animals tolerant of peanut. And a large study suggested that wheat allergy was more common among infants who hadn't eaten cereal until after 6 months of age.

The lower rates of peanut allergy in Israel could have been genetic. But Lack didn't think that explanation was plausible; he worked with a large Jewish population in London who shared the same genetic origin as Israelis. Perhaps it was due to lower rates of asthma, eczema, and allergic rhinitis (more commonly known as hay fever). Or perhaps it was due to early introduction of peanuts by mouth.

So in the mid-2000s, Lack, joined by George du Toit, Yitzhak Katz, and others, designed a study to clarify the matter. They decided to compare peanut allergy rates among groups of Jewish children in Israel and the UK in order to both pinpoint the prevalence of the condition and parse the connection between how often infants developed peanut allergy and how often their mothers ate peanuts. Their similar genetic background would rule out DNA as a factor.

And both countries had high levels of asthma, making that factor equal, too.

The study relied on questionnaires. One collected information on 8,826 children from thirteen schools in the UK and eleven in Israel regarding allergies to milk, eggs, sesame, peanut, and tree nuts, along with other allergic diseases. The other surveyed 176 mothers (99 from Israel and 77 from the UK) of babies up to 24 months old about when their child first ate peanuts, how often they ate them (along with sesame and other solid foods), and in what quantities.

Lack and his colleagues reported their findings in 2008. Peanut allergy was far more prevalent in the UK than in Israel—1.85 percent versus 0.17 percent. These percentages translate to relatively small numbers, but it's the difference that matters here: the allergy was ten times more common in the UK than in Israel. Sesame, tree nut, and egg allergies were also dramatically more common in the UK. Infants began eating egg, soy, wheat, vegetables, and fruit at around the same time in both countries. But the questionnaires revealed a striking difference in the timings of peanut introduction. "By 9 months of age, 69% of Israelis were eating peanut compared with only 10% of UK infants," the authors wrote. The Israeli children consumed an average of 7.1 grams of peanut protein during their first year of life, compared to 0 grams among the British children during that time frame. Nursing mothers in the UK ate far less peanut than their Israeli counterparts.

The data drove the researchers toward the compelling conclusion that eating peanuts early in life leads to fewer cases of peanut allergy among the Israeli children. The authors acknowledged that roasting peanuts may make them more allergenic, but realized that this couldn't explain the difference, because most of the peanut-containing foods that children eat in both countries use the roasted version. Social class could not explain the difference between the groups, nor could ancestry or the presence of other allergic diseases. Lack and his team knew the implications of their results: "Our study findings raise the question of whether early introduction rather than avoidance of peanut in infancy is the better strategy for prevention of [peanut allergy]," they wrote. At issue wasn't just whether delayed introduction had led to more cases of food allergy instead of fewer, but also whether taking the exact opposite tack was having the exact opposite effect.

THE BOLD NEXT STEP

With those results in hand, Lack and a team of researchers in the UK and the United States decided that the time had come to put the theory to the test. They started the Learning Early About Peanut Allergy (LEAP) trial to see if introducing peanuts into the diet early in life could prevent the allergy. They wanted to test whether early introduction would stop the allergy from developing in the first place and also whether it would curtail it in older children who were already allergic.

The only way to truly determine whether early introduction prevented food allergy was to compare two groups: one in which infants ate peanuts and one in which they didn't. That meant a randomized study. Lack knew that a rigorous trial was the only way to change minds regarding the practice of delaying the introduction of common allergens. The fear of giving babies peanuts had become so ingrained in many countries that even the medical authorities reversing their guidelines wasn't enough to persuade parents to try early introduction. They needed more data—and with the Immune Tolerance Network (ITN), the NIAID, and FARE providing the funding, the LEAP trial was about to provide it.

Beginning in December 2006, the LEAP team randomized 640 infants between 4 months and 11 months old to various treatment arms. All of the infants had severe eczema, egg allergy, or both—conditions that put them at high risk of peanut allergy. Among the 542 infants who tested negative for peanut allergy, 270 would be avoiding peanuts for the first two years of life. The other 272 would be eating a small amount of peanut protein every week for at least half of the weeks during the study. For the 98 infants who tested positive for peanut allergy with a skin prick test, 51 would be avoiding peanut and 47 would not. The plan was to follow the designated regimen until the children reached 60 months of age; more than 98 percent of them reached that goal, with just a few families withdrawing; some missing data and losing contact accounted for the remainder. The researchers eventually had to exclude data from an additional 20 infants because their families hadn't stuck to the protocol. That left 245 nonallergic and 50 allergic infants who avoided peanut and 255 nonallergic and 39 allergic infants who ate peanut.

After five years, it was time to see whether early introduction made a difference. If Lack's hunch was correct, then the number of infants with peanut allergy would be lower in the group who ate peanuts starting at the time they entered the study compared to the group who remained unexposed to peanuts. To find out, they turned to an oral food challenge, the most rigorous method to test for allergies.

First, the researchers also had to be certain that families had stuck with their designated protocol throughout the duration of the study. Parents had completed questionnaires about peanut consumption throughout the study. According to these reports, the infants in the peanut-eating group ate about 7.7 grams per week, and the infants in the no-peanut group ate 0 grams per week. The researchers corroborated the questionnaires by checking beds for peanut dust when the infants reached the 60-month mark. Among 423 beds out of the original 640 infants enrolled in the study, they found only about 4.1 micrograms of peanut per gram of dust in the beds of the peanut-avoiding group and about 91 micrograms in the beds of the peanut-consuming group. In other words, they could trust the data the families had provided.

Assured that the randomized infants represented early and delayed introduction, the researchers proceeded with oral food challenges for more than 96 percent of the participants. The results were stark. Among the infants who did not test positive for peanut allergy at the outset of the study, the incidence of this allergy was 86 percent less among those who consumed peanuts compared to those who did not by the time the children were 5 years old. Interestingly, the infants who had started out as positive for peanut allergy showed a similar pattern. By the time they were 5 years old, the children who consumed peanuts had a 70 percent reduction in this allergy compared to the children who avoided peanuts.

Other signs also showed the difference. Children in the avoidance group had larger wheals—the red circles from a skin prick test—and much higher levels of IgE antibodies targeted against peanut protein. Levels of IgG4, an immune system cell thought to be protective against food allergy, were higher among the early-introduction group, although the researchers emphasized that this finding doesn't mean that IgG4 caused those infants to not develop peanut allergy. The singular weakness of the study is the absence of a placebo arm; it would have been interesting to see rates of peanut allergy among a group of infants who consumed something, without the parents knowing whether or not it was peanut protein. Also, a baseline measurement of peanut dust in the homes of the participants, rather than only at 60 months, would have been useful.

But even with these limitations, the study undoubtedly confirmed what earlier data had hinted at. "Several years ago, we found that the risk of the development of peanut allergy was 10 times as high among Jewish children in the United Kingdom as it was in Israeli children of similar ancestry," the LEAP authors wrote in their study, published in *The New England Journal of Medicine* in early 2015. "The LEAP study showed that early oral introduction of peanuts could prevent allergy in high-risk sensitized infants and in nonsensitized infants." In addition, peanut avoidance was linked to a higher rate of peanut allergy compared to peanut consumption. That finding, they concluded, "raises questions about the usefulness of deliberate avoidance of peanuts as a strategy to prevent food allergy." The threads of observation that had started with egg-allergic mice in Denver years earlier had finally led to a stunning revelation. "I kick myself at times for not having put together the pieces earlier," says Lack.

It didn't take long for health authorities to realize what Lack and his team had discovered. By the end of August 2015, the American

Academy of Pediatrics had reversed course. Whereas the Academy had once recommended withholding peanut to prevent allergy among infants at high risk of the disease, now that no longer made sense. Instead, the Academy joined medical organizations from Australia, Canada, Europe, Japan, and Israel, among others, in a consensus statement that recommended early introduction of peanut to high-risk infants in countries where peanut allergy is prevalent. "Delaying the introduction of peanut can be associated with an increased risk of peanut allergy," the statement noted. The revelation also seeped into mainstream consciousness. Hugh Sampson, a pediatric allergist at Mount Sinai Hospital in New York, offered his independent assessment of the study to *The Washington Post*, noting that the LEAP trial, "showed you can prevent the development of peanut allergy."

But Lack and his colleagues knew this wasn't the end of the story. They had to know if the tolerance to peanuts lasted. A lower peanut allergy rate when children were 5 years old didn't mean anything if they developed the disease by age 6. And so they proceeded with the LEAP-ON study (for "Persistence of Oral Tolerance to Peanut") to see if children in the original study were still able to eat peanuts 12 months later.

A total of 556 of the original participants—282 from the original avoidance group and 274 from the peanut-consumption group—agreed to join LEAP-ON. They had one singular task: avoid peanut for the next twelve months. This time, there were more dropouts, with 223 of the 282 avoiders managing to keep peanut out of their diets for a full year and 127 of 274 of the peanut eaters doing so (perhaps many of the children in this group had grown to love peanut too much to skip it for a full year).

The results, published in *The New England Journal of Medicine* in 2016, validated the benefit of eating peanuts before 1 year of age. Among the original peanut-avoiding group, 18.6 percent had peanut allergy at 6 years old. And in the original peanut-consuming group, 4.8 percent had peanut allergy by that age. The researchers examined the data from several different angles and came to the conclusion that after a year of peanut abstinence following the LEAP study, peanut allergy was 74 percent less prevalent among children who'd consumed peanut early compared to those who hadn't. The LEAP and LEAP-ON studies, the researchers concluded, "show that 4 years of consuming peanut was sufficient to induce stable unresponsiveness to peanut." Of course the question of whether that tolerance would remain for years to come, even into adulthood, remained to be seen. But the fact was that early introduction rendered the majority of the children safe from peanut harm's way for the time being. Infants in the control group—those who did not start eating potential allergens early—developed more food allergies than the infants in the early-introduction group.

And it wasn't just peanuts. Another study, known as Enquiring About Tolerance (EAT), also by Lack's group and published just weeks after LEAP-ON, investigated whether infants could be safely introduced to multiple foods within the first few months of life. The team randomly assigned 1,303 3-month-old infants to breastfeeding plus a series of allergenic foods (milk, peanut, egg, sesame, fish, and wheat) or breastfeeding alone until they were 6 months old. By 5 months, the allergens proved safe among infants in the experimental group who ate the foods regularly; they also continued to nurse. Importantly, the LEAP and EAT researchers had wondered at the outset of this work whether consuming one potential allergen would confer protection against another—that eating fish, for example, could prevent shrimp allergy. That phenomenon turned out not to be the case; each specific food had to be consumed to be able to prevent that specific allergy.

The science suggesting a protective effect of early introduction of peanut was so strong that NIAID convened a panel of thirty experts to develop new recommendations for preventing peanut allergy. Just like the American Academy of Pediatrics, this panel, too, embraced early introduction.

The guidelines, still the most recent set issued by the NIAID, recommend that infants at high risk of peanut allergy (defined as having a close family history of the condition) start eating peanut-containing food between 4 and 6 months of age. Peanuts shouldn't be the first food, but they should be added to an infant's repertoire early on.

The NIAID guidelines also emphasized that when it came to other foods and prevention, more studies were needed. At our clinic at Stanford, we began advising parents and guardians to introduce potential allergens early in healthy infants regardless of whether they had eczema or a family history of food allergy (in other words, regardless of risk). We reasoned that exposing a child to potentially allergenic foods early and regularly, starting at around 4 to 6 months of age, would lower their chances of developing a food allergy. We suggested feeding babies a small serving of a powder containing ten to fifteen food allergens every day. Just a bit of each allergen, about 30 milligrams, was enough to see changes in the blood indicating a healthy tolerance of each food. Oral food challenges confirmed that this preventive measure worked. And the children had no side effects from these low doses.

After her first son developed allergies to tree nuts, peanuts, all seeds, egg, and nut-based oils, Jessica Frank thought hard about introducing these foods to her second child. "We had a lot of conversations with our pediatrician and our allergist," she recalls. Frank and her husband wondered if early introduction would protect their newborn from the food allergies that had hit their firstborn so severely. "If we wait two or three years, will his body become allergic to foods?" she remembers wondering. At the same time, having seen what those allergens triggered in their first child, they fretted about intentionally exposing their younger child to the same symptoms.

Their local allergist encouraged them to go for it, reassuring them that if their second son had a reaction, they'd know how to handle it—after all, they were experienced food allergy parents now. Making sure their older son wasn't around in order to reduce the risk of accidental exposure, Frank and her husband gave their younger son some Bamba, an Israeli snack food made with peanuts that's often given to babies (and used in the LEAP study) when he was about 10 months old. He didn't react. Soon they offered him cashews. Again he had no reaction. Then came almond butter. "Our second son was introduced to all the nuts before he was even a year old," says Frank. He remains free from all allergies—including seasonal ones, Frank notes. She can't say for sure that early introduction made the difference, but she knows it may have played a part. "We were confident in our choice," she says, "and I'm really glad that we did it earlier rather than later."

NOT JUST PEANUTS

The striking results of the EAT, LEAP, and LEAP-ON studies led to the question of whether early introduction works for preventing other common food allergies, too. Egg is a logical choice to tackle, and several studies have done so. A Japanese study called Prevention of Egg Allergy with Tiny Amounts (PETIT) looked at early egg introduction by randomizing 147 infants, starting between 4 and 5 months of age, to consume either heated egg powder every day or a placebo. They also received aggressive eczema treatment. The study was ended after an analysis of 100 patients done midstream showed the power of early introduction. Egg allergy developed among 4 of the 47 children in the egg-consuming group and 18 of the 47 children in the egg-avoiding group (data from 6 of the 100 couldn't be included in the analysis). PETIT wasn't all smooth sailing; 6 of the children randomized to the egg-eating group had to be hospitalized for an allergic reaction versus none in the placebo group.

In 2013, researchers from Australia and Sweden reported their study, known as Solids Timing for Allergy Research (STAR), investigating whether egg exposure could reduce the allergy in infants with eczema. In a blind, randomized trial, 49 infants had a teaspoon of raw whole egg powder and 37 infants had a teaspoon of rice powder daily for four months, starting at 4 months of age. Both groups had cooked eggs starting at 8 months old. At the outset of the study, a third of all the babies enrolled showed early signs of egg allergy (in the form of anti-egg antibodies) when they were 4 months old. But by the time the infants were 1 year old, the researchers saw fewer cases of egg allergy in the egg-consuming group compared to the rice powder group. Although the difference in this study was slight, the researchers deduced that regular oral egg exposure could desensitize high-risk infants to egg.

In the Beating Egg Allergy Trial (BEAT), one of the largest studies on early introduction of egg, researchers in Australia and the UK randomized 319 infants who were not allergic to egg but had at least one immediate family member with egg allergy to a regimen of either egg powder or rice powder from 4 months to 8 months of age. Importantly, 14 of the children on the egg-powder arm reacted to the food and had to stop the treatment after a week. Subtracting those participants and others who stopped the trial left 254 children for the duration of the study. When they were 1 year old, 20 percent of the rice powder group and 11 percent of the egg group were reactive to egg white. The egg powder, it seemed, had reduced the development of allergy.

Not every study looking at early egg introduction has delivered favorable results, though. The Hen's Egg Allergy Prevention (HEAP) study randomized 383 infants who were not allergic to egg to consume either egg white powder (184 children) or a placebo (199 children) three times per week starting between 4 and 6 months of age until they were 1 year old. At the end of the study, 5.6 percent of the intervention group had egg sensitivity compared to 2.6 percent of the placebo group. The international group of authors also deemed the approach unsafe because nearly 6 percent of the infants they initially screened for the study already had egg allergy. Starting a prevention strategy at 4 to 6 months of age was already too late for these infants, the authors noted.

Given the conflicting findings, a meta-analysis—a study of studies—is helpful for figuring out where the balance of evidence lies. A group of UK researchers took up that task in 2016. Five trials provided moderate-certainty evidence that introducing egg when babies are 4 to 6 months old reduces the chances that they will develop an egg allergy. The data may not be as strong as they were in the LEAP and LEAP-ON studies, but the approach is trustworthy.

KEY STUDIES ON EARLY INTRODUCTION OF FOOD ALLERGENS

STUDY NAME	YEAR	COUNTRY	AGES	NUMBER OF PARTICIPANTS (TREATMENT/ PLACEBO)	CONCLUSION
EGG					
Prevention of Egg Allergy with Tiny Amount Intake Trial (PETIT)	2017	Japan	4 to 5 months	147 (73/74)	Gradual introduction of heated egg along with aggressive eczema treatment safely prevents egg allergy in high-risk* infants.
Beating Egg Allergy Trial (BEAT)	2017	Australia and UK	4 months	319 (165/154)	Whole-egg powder reduced sensitivity to egg whites among high-risk infants, although 8.5 percent of infants in the study could not complete the treatment.
Starting Time of Egg Protein (STEP)	2017	Australia	4 to 6 months	820 (407/413)	Infants at high risk of egg allergy (no eczema but parent with allergy) did not have substantially lower rates of egg allergy by 1 year of age when they ate eggs between 4 and 6 months of age.

STUDY NAME	YEAR	COUNTRY	AGES	NUMBER OF PARTICIPANTS (TREATMENT/ PLACEBO)	CONCLUSION
Hen's Egg Allergy Prevention (HEAP)	2017	Germany	4 to 6 months	383 (184/199)	Consuming egg starting at 4 to 6 months of age prevents egg sensitization or allergy. Many infants were already allergic to egg when they enrolled in the study at 4 months old, indicating that delayed introduction was not the sole problem.
Solids Timing for Allergy Research (STAR)	2013	Australia	4 months	86 (49/37)	Regular, early egg exposure led to immune system tolerance and a reduction in egg allergy among infants with eczema. Caution must be taken with these high-risk infants, many of whom are already allergic to egg by 4 months of age.
MULTIPLE FOODS					
Enquiring About Tolerance (EAT)	2016	UK	3 months	1,303 (652 early introduction/651 standard introduction)	By 5 months of age, infants in the early introduction group were eating all allergens included in the study. A separate analysis did not confirm the benefit of early introduction, raising questions about the best "dose" of food to give early on.

STUDY NAME	YEAR	COUNTRY	AGES	NUMBER OF PARTICIPANTS (TREATMENT/ PLACEBO)	CONCLUSION
PEANUTS					
Learning Early About Peanut Allergy (LEAP)	2015	UK	4 to 11 months	640 (319/321)	Early introduction of peanuts resulted in lower rates of peanut allergy among high-risk children.

*High risk is defined as having eczema and/or one or both parents with the food allergy in question.

That being said, parents should always exercise caution when it comes to introducing potential allergens, especially when an infant has eczema, other food allergies, or close relatives with food allergy. Which brings us to . . .

HOW TO INTRODUCE POTENTIAL ALLERGENS EARLY

A word of caution before discussing how to introduce new foods: **Parents who are concerned that their child may have a food allergy must absolutely consult a pediatrician and/or a pediatric allergist before introducing solid foods.** Access to immediate, up-to-date, and live input from a nearby medical professional may be vital to your child's health. And consulting with your doctor will ensure that your child is on his or her radar as a potential allergy sufferer.

This overview is not intended to be prescriptive. Rather, it offers a glimpse of the landscape of early introduction, so that parents are equipped with the necessary references for making informed decisions about their family. Although medical professionals are a crucial part of the equation, your own knowledge will also help light the way ahead.

Allergic reactions are almost always easy to spot. Although it can feel alarming, especially due to scary news stories, early introduction is nothing to fear. Whatever trepidation parents may feel at the outset can be allayed by the knowledge that the evidence supporting early introduction is substantial and sound. The American Academy of Pediatrics, the European Academy of Allergy and Clinical Immunology, the American Academy of Allergy, Asthma, and Immunology, the Australasian Society of Clinical Immunology and Allergy, the National Institute of Allergy and Infectious Diseases—all of these agencies and others have issued food allergy guidelines that include early introduction.

Signs of an Allergy

Knowing what to look for can help. The first key is being aware of *when* to look—symptoms can appear up to two hours after eating an allergen. The appearance of a rash or hives around the mouth or face may indicate a mild allergic reaction. Albeit extremely rare, severe symptoms include nonstop vomiting, respiratory issues like repeated coughing, difficulty breathing, or sudden lethargy. The chances of a life-threatening reaction are exceedingly rare. **If a child develops any of these more concerning symptoms after trying a new food, seek medical attention immediately.**

As you introduce new foods to your child, it may also help to remember that eating solid food is part of our natural development. Food is part of our survival, and enjoying and sharing it is part of what makes us human. Watching a baby delight in a sweet fruit or a savory bite of cheese is part of the fun of parenting. Every new taste is a little gift.

When to Start

As discussed earlier, the research to date suggests that babies should be exclusively breastfed if possible, formula-fed, or a combination of both until at least 4 months of age. Wait until this time to introduce your infant to solid foods. There's plenty of guidance available, whether through your pediatrician or your favorite book on infant health, on the signs that indicate a baby is ready for solid food.

Sitting without help and reaching for food are good indicators that your baby wants to try solid foods. Overlapping the introduction of solid foods with breastfeeding is ideal. Babies still depend on these first forms of nourishment until they are ingesting enough solid food for a completely nutritious diet. There is also some evidence that continuing to breastfeed (if possible) may reduce the risk of food allergy from newly introduced foods.

Does your infant have good neck control? Are they interested in food? Do they open their mouths when you offer food on a spoon? If the answer to these questions is yes, then your baby is likely ready to begin the sensory adventure that is solid food.

It's a good idea to introduce babies to diverse foods. If you can share meals as a family, an infant in the process of experiencing solid foods for the first time will want to have what everyone else is having. And it makes putting dinner on the table that much easier.

A More Detailed Look

New foods can be introduced while an adult is present, mostly to watch swallowing and protect against choking. Remember, allergic reactions are incredibly rare, and when they do occur in infants, they are typically very mild. Keeping the baby upright eases swallowing.

After offering a small taste of a prepared serving of a single or mixed food, the adult can offer the rest of the serving. And you don't have to introduce foods one at a time; there's no evidence supporting that approach. If you suspect your baby may be having an allergic reaction (again, these events are rare), consult a board-certified allergist who can test for allergies to a variety of foods—a practice that again underscores the fact that it's safe to introduce many at once.

For babies who are less than 6 months old, new foods should be mashed or pureed. By 8 or 9 months, babies can eat lumpy foods. Small pieces of solid but soft foods can be served on a high chair tray or plate. By 12 months, babies can eat solid foods cut into small pieces. Foods that are rich in iron are good to introduce early. These include fortified cereals, well-cooked eggs, tofu, legumes, and proteins including meat, fish, and poultry.

The Importance of Diet Diversity

When it comes to infant diets, variety isn't just the spice of life; it's essential. A 2014 analysis of data from a European study called Protection Against Allergy: Study in Rural Environments (PASTURE), which included 856 children, found that those with more diverse diets during their first year of life tended to have fewer food allergies regardless of whether they were at high or low risk for food allergies. By the time they're about a year old, babies should be eating cereals (wheat or rice, typically), a range of fruits and vegetables, dairy, and meat or meat alternatives.

Contrary to the approach many caregivers tend to take, new foods do not need to be introduced one at a time. In fact, it's better to introduce several foods at once. The more types of protein the gut is exposed to, the more tolerant it will be of new ones.

At Stanford, we typically recommend that tree nuts, legumes (soy and peanut), milk, wheat, and egg be introduced into the diet early, whenever a baby is ready for solid foods. Serving sizes don't need to be large. In fact, we have found that smaller serving sizes are better tolerated, pose fewer safety issues, and are just as effective as large portions at expanding the variety of foods without triggering reactions. A dietician or allergist can suggest options for preparing these foods, but obviously the main importance is that they be easily consumed by a baby without teeth and unaccustomed to chewing. With all we now know, it's time to shed the outdated practices of introducing foods one at a time with several days between and of holding off on feeding a baby a particular food because it's thought to be a common allergen.

PROBIOTICS AND PREBIOTICS

Pro- and prebiotic supplements aren't foods. However, they warrant a mention here because of their increasing presence in health food and vitamin stores. Parents may be tempted to turn to these products to help their children grow a healthy microbiome.

Nursing mothers should not supplement their diets with probiotics or prebiotics in the hope of preventing food allergy in their babies. An expert panel convened by the American Academy of Allergy, Asthma, and Immunology, the EAACI, and other groups found insufficient evidence of any benefit from this approach.

Investigations of whether children who take these supplements have a lower risk of food allergy haven't shown a benefit, but the studies also have not been powerful enough to provide a clear reading. Prebiotics may reduce eczema, which can in turn help prevent food allergy, but again, the data are still inconsistent at this time. Families concerned about milk allergy should be aware that these supplements sometimes contain milk proteins.

Food allergy research is advancing faster than ever, and that includes the science of early introduction. Future years may bring more specific regimens for first foods, bolstered by increasing knowledge about how our immune systems take shape and how genetics, nutrients, and the environment influence that process. We are also seeing the emergence of products (covered in a later chapter) to make early introduction easy, helping parents make sure that their children are exposed to common allergens at an ideal time and in ideal amounts. But wherever food allergy is headed, we know that avoidance is not the way toward prevention. With all the areas to explore in this ever-expanding landscape, it's nice to know the places we don't need to visit again.

THE BOTTOM LINE

- Current evidence suggests that early exposure to common food allergens prevents food allergy regardless of risk.

- Babies should start on a diverse diet early and often, beginning at around 4 to 6 months of age.

- If a child already has a diagnosed food allergy, consult with a board-certified allergist before starting solid food introduction.

- Recent guidelines recommend introducing potentially allergenic foods regularly after 4 to 6 months of exclusive breastfeeding.

- Be watchful of symptoms when introducing new foods.

- There is no need to introduce foods one at a time.

- Testing by a board-certified allergist should follow any reaction that arises.

Chapter 7

BEYOND AVOIDANCE: THE BRAVE NEW WORLD OF IMMUNOTHERAPY

The pioneering work to retrain the immune system and end the suffering

Kim Yates's daughter, Tessa Grosso, was born with more than fifteen allergies, including dairy, shellfish, and eggs. The first of Tessa's many trips to the emergency room came after she ate a single Goldfish cracker when she was 9 months old. When she was just short of 3 years old, she vomited after milk spilled on her arms. Rye bread that turned out to have traces of dairy and wheat once sent her into anaphylaxis. One of her worst allergic episodes occurred at a restaurant they'd come to depend on as a safe place. The cooks swapped their regular rice noodles for wheat without telling the customers. Tessa left in an ambulance. She survived, but the event left Kim more desperate than ever. "There has to be a better way," she decided.

Early introduction of common allergens is an excellent approach for families wishing to prevent food allergy. But it doesn't help the more than 60 million people around the world living with the disease. For so many parents, the fear of offering an infant that first tiny bite of egg pales in comparison to the fear of a peanut-allergic elementary school student on a class trip or a wheat-allergic teenager heading to a friend's house on pizza-making night. And while parents suffer the tangled knot of worry, food-allergic children must learn to navigate a world where danger lurks in every corner and where even the most vigilant sentry cannot stop an enemy from slipping past. Food allergy is burdensome. It's stressful. It can leave a child feeling left out or stigmatized. It can leave parents fretting and overprotective. It can leave newly diagnosed adults coping with an unexpected late-life transformation. It's entirely possible to adjust to life with food allergy. But given the choice, most people would rather just live without it.

That brings us to the heart of the new era of food allergy care and the emergence of treatments capable of reversing the condition. Alongside the movement toward early introduction, pioneering researchers around the world have been revolutionizing the treatment of food allergy by reeducating the immune system, slowly but surely. The approach, known as oral immunotherapy, is rapidly evolving into a concrete, accessible program that is transforming the lives of people living with food allergy. And it's at the forefront of a steady flow of exciting new options that are pushing open the floodgates and truly changing the world of food allergy for the better.

This chapter explains how immunotherapy works and lays out the evidence for its benefit. Following the evolution of the research, we look at the small early studies that hinted at the power of immunotherapy (IT), and one type of immunotherapy in particular, oral immunotherapy (OIT). Powerful randomized controlled trials confirmed the benefit of IT and refined the process; studies paired OIT with biologic drugs, a combination that has expanded the benefit even further. We'll also look at the entirety of immunotherapy, which includes sublingual immunotherapy (SLIT) and epicutaneous immunotherapy (EPIT, also known as patch therapy), approaches that have also yielded meaningful results, though with somewhat different mechanisms. This massive amount of data—and the help it offers to food allergy sufferers—owes a debt to the thousands of brave patients and families who have participated in clinical trials over the past few decades. Whatever benefit these individuals may have received for themselves, their contribution to the field is incalculable.

By the time you finish reading this chapter, you will be well versed in the research behind immunotherapy as a program to reverse food allergy. These studies (and many others we don't have room to include) are the foundation on which this new era stands. Think of this chapter as a guidebook. You don't need to know everything about a country in order to get the most out of your trip there, but the more knowledge you have, the more sure you can be about your decisions.

A brief word about clinical trials: These studies are how researchers rigorously test experimental treatments. They typically proceed in three phases. Phase 1 trials are small studies aimed at testing a new drug or other intervention for safety. Phase 2 trials are larger, though usually conducted at a single institution. They enable researchers to gauge whether the treatment warrants a large, costly investigation. Phase 3 trials are those large, costly investigations. These studies are often run at multiple centers and involve many patients. Phase 3 trials compare experimental treatments with standard approaches by randomly assigning patients to one or the other (or a placebo, if no standard intervention exists). Patients usually don't know which treatment they're receiving, and the same goes for the investigators leading the study, a measure that helps reduce any bias in the results. When a phase 2 or 3 study is double-blind and randomized, it means that no one knows which patients received which treatment and the treatment assignments were left to chance. Phase 3 trials provide the necessary evidence for a drug to be approved for widespread use.

WHAT IS IMMUNOTHERAPY?

The concept of immunotherapy, or IT, has actually been around for some time. Remember that 1908 case, from chapter 5, in which Alfred Schofield cured a 13-year-old boy of egg allergy by feeding him minuscule but increasing amount of egg over six months? That was oral immunotherapy, also called OIT. The approach is a form of desensitization, a phenomenon that humanity has taken advantage of for centuries. History tells us that King Mithridates VI, who ruled northern Anatolia from 120 to 63 BC, concocted a potion that included tiny amounts of arsenic and various venoms as a way to desensitize his body to the poisons he thought his enemies might use on him. The practice of desensitizing people with respiratory allergies with shots of medication began in 1911. However, it's only in the past few decades that immunologists have turned substantial attention to puzzling out whether IT works for food allergy, and if so, how exactly it should be done.

The science of IT is rooted in the immune mechanisms that drive food allergy to develop in the first place. As earlier chapters have described, the immune system triggers allergic reactions to food when it mistakes a protein in the food for something harmful. For reasons that research is still unraveling—delayed exposure to a food, introduction of food proteins through skin that is dry or has eczema rather than through the mouth, an overly sanitized environment, overuse of antibiotics, and other possibilities—the immune system creates a type of antibody known as IgE, specifically trained against a food protein. Once peanut-specific or egg-specific or sesame-specific IgE exists, the immune system will catapult those antibodies into action every time these proteins enter the body. The mobilized IgE antibodies adhere to structures on the food protein known as antigens. That connection is like turning the key in the ignition, spurring a host of reactions all designed to eliminate the problem. But because the problem isn't real, the reactions hurt the person instead. The nitty-gritty details of the processes taking place in the immune system that render a person intolerant of one food or another are innumerable and complicated. However, research has found that a sufficient presence of protein-specific IgE is a fairly reliable indicator that an individual is allergic to the food containing that protein.

The basic principle underlying IT is that the immune system can be retrained so that it stops producing those food-specific IgE antibodies when the proteins appear. Laboratory researchers are actively grappling with the exact details of how that reversal occurs. The evidence so far suggests that the slow introduction of tiny amounts of allergens triggers the production of another type of anti-body called IgG4. Studies of IT to treat peanut allergy have found a notable increase in IgG4. IgG4 antibodies compete with IgE to reach the target protein. If the IgG4 antibody lands on the protein antigen first, then IgE has no room. Without that contact, the cascade of events that culminates in anaphylaxis never gets started. IgG4 antibodies don't launch an attack; they block one. IT also appears to increase the number of regulatory T cells, also called Tregs, which help regulate the immune system and prevent autoimmune diseases, a category of ailments that have been linked to food allergy. IT also appears to decrease the amount of T helper type 2, or Th2, cells, another piece of the immune factory that becomes dysfunctional when food allergy arises.

Of course it's not necessary to understand how the immune system recalibrates itself during IT in order for the process to work. At Stanford University alone, thousands of children and adults have undergone treatment that has aimed to provide a life free from the fear of a severe allergic reaction. Kari and her team have spent the last fifteen years investigating the ideal IT regimens for a wide range of situations—peanut allergy; milk allergy; allergies to several foods at once; allergies with and without asthma; adult-onset food allergy; allergies with and without eosinophilic esophagitis—in order to identify the program with the best chance of converting someone from allergic to nonallergic as safely, permanently, and quickly as possible. Many people who have gone through IT are able to tolerate accidental exposure with the allergen without any reaction. Others reach the point where they can freely eat the allergen just like any other food. Either way, it's life-changing. More on that up ahead.

THE ERA OF IMMUNOTHERAPY
RESEARCH BEGINS

As we described in chapter 5, the twists and turns of food allergy research during the early twentieth century cast oral immunotherapy largely to the sidelines. In the 1980s, something changed: food allergy rates began increasing. We now know that this rise led to recommendations centered on delayed introduction, which likely perpetuated the problem. Treatment options were nonexistent. Doctors and allergists had one counsel to offer, and that was to avoid the food allergen. The reasoning was sound. Don't eat the food and you won't have to worry about having an allergic reaction to it. But obviously that approach couldn't stop a restaurant cook from switching rice noodles to wheat noodles without telling a wheat-allergic customer or a packaged food maker from failing to list sesame in the ingredients. It couldn't account for someone allergic to milk buying toothpaste that (who knows why) contained that very ingredient. In other words, it couldn't account for life. And even if people could avoid an allergen for their entire life, should they have to? What if there was another way?

In the early 1970s, an Italian allergist named Giampiero Patriarca was studying drug allergies. He wanted to know what was happening in the immune system that could make someone allergic to a particular chemical—and whether there was anything to be done about it. Drug allergies could be a problem by preventing someone from taking a crucial antibiotic or a diagnostic test. Based on what his research suggested about the biological pathways responsible for allergies, Patriarca thought it might be possible for someone to become desensitized. He published several case studies charting his attempts and successes.

The encouraging results eventually turned Patriarca's mind to food allergy. In 1984, he and his team tested a desensitization treatment on nineteen people with a range of single food allergies—milk, egg, fish, and orange. The approach, the researchers wrote in the publication of their work, "was successful in 14 out of 15 patients who followed it correctly." The benefit didn't last, however. Within twelve months, all fourteen patients were allergic again. Also, this was a case report, a type of study that provides an intriguing anecdote but doesn't offer rigorous data to the broader investigation of an experimental treatment.

The first substantial trial came in the late 1990s. By this time, desensitization was part and parcel of the treatment for respiratory allergy. People with asthma and hay fever commonly sought routine allergy shots to block wrongly trained antibodies. But oral immunotherapy—consuming a food allergen—hadn't kept pace. Most allergists still believed the only option was keeping the food out of the diet. In 1992, a group of researchers from Colorado published a study of eleven people with peanut allergy randomized to receive a treatment consisting of injections of peanut extract or no treatment at all. They started with a small amount of extract and slowly scaled up the amount of protein, which they then gave weekly for a year. After six weeks and then at the end of the study, the researchers conducted oral food challenges, giving all the participants a small amount of peanut to see if the treatment improved tolerance. The results were mixed. Participants receiving peanut extract tolerated peanut better at the end of the study than at the beginning. The wheals that appeared during skin prick tests became smaller. The no-treatment group showed neither of these changes. The participants receiving the injections still had allergic reactions, often requiring epinephrine to quell, but it took higher quantities of the allergen to trigger that response. Three of the six patients on the experimental arm could handle weekly injections for the full year. The researchers knew the approach was promising, but the best regimen for future studies remained unclear. This study used the subcutaneous route, sending the allergen into the body through an injection rather than by eating it. The results, combined with the findings of a 1992 study of subcutaneous immunotherapy in which one participant died due to a pharmaceutical error, left researchers with the sense that this route wasn't safe. Subcutaneous immunotherapy was abandoned.

FOCUSING ON THE ORAL ROUTE

Within a few years, however, researchers were warming to the idea that offering nearly microscopic amounts of a food, with gradual but consistent increases over a prolonged amount of time, might have a dramatic effect on an allergy. A small and careful approach with a big result—that was the goal.

Patriarca and his group returned to the medical literature in 1998 with a more formal study. This time, they treated fourteen cases of food allergy (six milk, five egg, two fish, and one apple) with a desensitization regimen and compared the results to ten similarly food-allergic people who stuck to avoidance. All of the patients on the treatment arm—which included taking small but increasing amounts of the culprit food by mouth—became desensitized. "All the treated patients are now able to tolerate any food with no untoward effects or need for preventive drugs," the authors wrote.

The results encouraged the team to go bigger. In 2003, they published results of a study in which 59 people with food allergy underwent oral desensitization. The researchers were addressing two questions in this study: Could the patients tolerate the treatment? How would it change their immune systems? According to their report, 48 of the 59 participants were able to complete the program. Their allergic reactions were mild, below the point of needing epinephrine. And their IgE levels declined, indicating a change at the source of the problem.

The next significant step forward came from Germany, with a study published in 2007. A group of researchers in Berlin randomly assigned a group of children with egg or milk allergy to either treatment with what the researchers called specific oral tolerance induction (SOTI) or a standard elimination diet. SOTI entailed taking their allergen at home daily following a prescribed regimen. Once they completed the SOTI regimen, which took about twenty-one months, those children then kept the food out of their diet for two months, at which point all the participants took an oral food challenge. Nine of the 25 SOTI children lost their allergy entirely. Three of them could tolerate the food as long as they continued to take a bit of it regularly. And for 4 of them, the allergy became less severe. Interestingly, 7 of the 20 children on the elimination diet could also tolerate their allergen at the end of the study, with the drop in IgE levels to match, perhaps due to their natural tolerance increasing. The authors saw an advantage for the SOTI arm, though. Those children had a higher threshold before an allergic reaction—they could eat more of the allergen—and the chance that they would have a severe reaction after eating the food accidentally was far reduced.

By this time, the dam had broken. Suddenly studies of immunotherapy poured into the medical literature at a steady clip. Every year brought new breakthroughs. And each new report brought reasons to feel encouraged about the future that IT had to offer.

Many studies focused on individual food allergies—namely, milk, egg, and peanut. These first studies sharpened the IT process into four basic steps. First, the researcher needs to figure out the highest dose of a food that a person can tolerate. Then the treatment begins, starting at the highest tolerated dose and gradually increasing to a maintenance dose that is identified at the start of the study. The third step is the maintenance stage, when the patient continues to take that maintenance dose for a period of time. Finally, an oral food challenge tests whether the patient's immune system can now tolerate the allergen. Often, studies include an additional phase when the patient stops taking the food altogether for a period of time in order to see whether the tolerance sticks.

Turning Food into Medicine

The use of the word *dose* here is important. In the context of OIT, food is actually used as medicine. Study participants aren't just eating a portion of food (however tiny that portion may be); they are taking medication. In OIT, the medications are the allergens, often in powdered forms that can be stirred into pudding or applesauce. They are kept in sterilized pantries and refrigerators that ensure the food is free from any other substance. Each dose is measured on a laboratory scale with exacting precision. Researchers who conduct OIT studies source the foods from specific outlets that ensure the item is free from contamination. At the Sean N. Parker Center for Allergy & Asthma Research, for example, we purchase cashew flour from a farm that grows only cashews, nothing else. Procedures like this are crucial to making sure that our data are reliable and reproducible. The quest to optimize OIT regimens for the full range of food allergy conditions demands the highest standards. The purpose of OIT clinical trials is to identify therapies that the FDA can approve, that clinics around the world can follow, and that insurance companies will cover. That means conducting studies with the same careful methodology as we see in studies for new cancer drugs or new diabetes treatments. OIT is a medical treatment.

Several studies of milk allergy delivered early encouraging results. For example, when researchers at Johns Hopkins University, led by Robert Wood, randomized 20 children to milk OIT or placebo, they found that milk OIT vastly improved the children's tolerance. On the very first day of treatment, the researchers identified each patient's starting dose, the threshold amount that triggered a reaction. By eight weeks, the dose was up to 500 milligrams, which the children maintained for three to four months (although one child dropped out of the study due to eczema resulting from the escalating dose). Importantly, this was the first OIT study to make the oral food challenge double-blind at the end of the treatment; neither the doctors nor the families knew whether a particular test result was from a child on the milk arm or the placebo arm. That practice helps eliminate any bias that might color how the child responds or how the physician interprets the results. At the end of the study, the 19 children who underwent milk OIT could tolerate an estimated 5,000 milligrams of milk protein before reacting, compared to an estimated 40 milligrams in the placebo group. The process wasn't without incidents. The milk OIT children did have some allergic reactions, although these consisted mostly of an itchy mouth or abdominal pain. Reactions with multiple symptoms, indicating a more severe allergy, were very rare.

Several other studies continued to propel OIT forward. Almost all of the sixty 2-year-old children in one study from Spain became fully desensitized to milk. Similarly, a study of milk-allergic schoolchildren in Finland found that almost all of the participants who were able to tolerate milk by the end of the study were still tolerant three years later. By the end of 2014, at least 278 milk-allergic children had been through OIT studies, with 84 percent becoming desensitized to their allergen by the end of their study. A group of researchers from Spain found that patients who had multiple allergies or a history of anaphylaxis might be at higher risk for severe allergic reactions during OIT trials, work that further helped investigators and patients know what to expect during these studies.

Like the early milk trials, the first egg OIT studies were small but encouraging. In a 2007 study of 7 children, all the participants tolerated more egg protein at the end of the study than at the start, and at a higher quantity than a person would typically be exposed to accidentally. In a 2010 study from Japan, 6 children between the ages of 7 and 12 years who had severe egg allergy underwent OIT treatment that left all of them desensitized. After a year, all 6 children could eat more than one egg with no reaction. A year later, a Spanish team reported their results of a study involving 23 egg-allergic children, ages 5 to 17. Twenty children reached the point of eating a whole cooked egg per day without any severe reactions, 14 of them within five days. Six months later, they could still tolerate eggs. By 2014, of the 165 children who participated in egg OIT studies, 81 percent (132 children) had become desensitized. And in 2017, a group from France reported that among 84 egg-allergic children randomized to avoidance or OIT, 25 of the OIT children reacted to egg during a food challenge at the end of the study, versus 40 of the avoidance children.

Of course many OIT researchers were eager to see if an immune system reactive to peanut could be reeducated. Stacie Jones at the University of Arkansas and Wesley Burks at the University of North Carolina were the first to design such a trial. Again, the initial stretch of studies gave reason to hope. In a small OIT study reported in 2009, 4 children had their peanut allergy completely disappear. All 4 could eat ten peanuts at the end of the study, a quantity that was up to 478 times higher than what they could tolerate at the start. In Arkansas, 20 out of 28 enrolled children between the ages of 1 and 16 grew to tolerate peanut in a study involving a dose of 300 milligrams of peanut flour given for up to two years. Nearly all the children could tolerate 3,900 milligrams of peanut protein without any symptoms by the end of the study.

A few years later, a group of international researchers banded together to better understand whether peanut OIT posed a danger. The team, based at five different centers in the United States and Israel, enrolled a total of 352 patients to an OIT regimen using peanuts, peanut butter, or peanut flour. Through a cumulative 240,351 doses, 95 allergic reactions were severe enough to require epinephrine. And 298 patients—85 percent—were able to tolerate the maintenance dose. The study made two points clear: first, that OIT could be an effective treatment for peanut allergy, and second, that OIT must be done by a medical professional at a healthcare facility. By the end of 2014, at least 516 peanut-allergic children had been treated with OIT and about 82 percent emerged from their studies desensitized.

THE LANDMARK TRIALS

The first years of intensive OIT research set the stage for the kind of clinical trials that medical care depends on. The only way doctors and families could know for sure whether the treatment worked was to see the results of randomized clinical trials comparing it to the standard approach of avoidance. The past few years have seen the completion of several landmark studies, and these are at the heart of the new world of food allergy care.

Among the most important of these trials was PALISADE, an abbreviation for Peanut Allergy Oral Immunotherapy Study of AR101 for Desensitization. AR101 is an OIT drug made of peanut protein flour, now approved by the FDA and marketed under the name Palforzia (we will refer to this drug as AR101 throughout this book). Even though AR101 is no different from other peanut powder used in OIT, its designation as a drug facilitates its use in studies and private treatment clinics. The PALISADE study was a huge international undertaking conducted by about 70 researchers, including the team at Stanford. Nearly 500 peanut-allergic children between the ages of 4 and 17 were randomized to receive either AR101 or a placebo. The dose escalated until the treatment arm reached 300 milligrams per day, which they continued to take for 24 weeks. The study was double-blind; the participants didn't know whether they were ingesting peanut protein or placebo, and neither did the researchers.

The goal of the study was to see how many participants on each arm could consume 600 milligrams or more of peanut without developing symptoms that would stop them from doing so. According to the results, published in *The New England Journal of Medicine* in 2018, the treatment had a dramatic effect. Of the 372 people randomized to the AR101 arm, 250 (67 percent) could ingest 600 milligrams or more of peanut protein with no serious reactions. By comparison, only 5 of the 124 people on the placebo arm (4 percent) could manage that feat. The treatment group had fewer severe symptoms during the final food challenge, but also fewer moderate and mild symptoms. It's important to note that although PALISADE was supported with a federal research grant, the study also received funding by Aimmune Therapeutics, the company that makes AR101. That doesn't make the data any less rigorous, but it's important to be aware of potential conflicts when we're looking at research studies.

Ronin Fisher joined our study when he was 5 years old. He'd been diagnosed with peanut allergy when he was 18 months old and vomited after eating peanut butter. His father, Masa, remembers how dramatically the diagnosis changed their lives. They enrolled their son in a nut-free day care and then preschool. They safeguarded their daily lives against an accidental run-in. They reminded their families before visits. "It's like you join the club," says Masa. Neither Ronin's family nor the study team knew whether he was actually consuming peanut powder once he started the study, but they were fully committed to the process regardless. After six months, Ronin was "unblinded"—it turned out he'd been on the peanut powder arm and could now tolerate 300 milligrams of peanut. He continued his dosing, now on the open-label portion of the study. Like some families, Ronin's parents weren't aiming for an allergy-free existence. "We're reducing the immune reaction rather than eliminating his allergy," says Masa. "We still carry epinephrine and ask about ingredients." And he worries about the years ahead when his son is a teenager managing his allergy independently. But they are relieved that Ronin can now better tolerate an accidental exposure to peanut, a result that has left Masa optimistic for the food allergy community as a whole. "This is a viable course for others with peanut allergy," he says.

Another bedrock study, known as POISED (Peanut Oral Immunotherapy Study: Safety, Efficacy, and Discovery), funded by the NIAID, looked at whether patients who become desensitized to peanut during the initial stage of a trial need to continue taking a "dose" of peanut afterward in order to stay desensitized. The trial, conducted by our team at Stanford University, enrolled 120 peanut-allergic people between the ages of 7 and 55. Ninety-five of these participants received a daily dose of peanut that escalated to 4 grams; the other 25 took a placebo made of oat flour. After two years, 84 percent of the treatment group could safely consume peanut protein, versus 4 percent of the placebo group.

Andrew Schatz, who had been diagnosed with multiple allergies when he was 1 year old, was among the children we treated in the peanut group. His immune system had come to tolerate milk and eggs as he grew up, but remained stubbornly opposed to peanuts. Because the allergy had been diagnosed through a test, Andrew had never been exposed to peanut until one day after school when he was play-wrestling with a friend. The friend had eaten peanut butter at lunch, and a bit of it must have remained on his clothes or his face. Andrew's lips swelled to three times their normal size. And that was just from being brushed with the protein; Andrew hadn't even swallowed it. His parents, Pete and Leilani, enrolled Andrew in the POISED trial soon afterward. The 4-milligram starting dose made Andrew's tongue tingle and itch. He went to the clinic every two weeks for two years so his dose could be gradually increased, eventually reaching 4 grams every day without concerning symptoms. These days he swallows a peanut at 10:15 P.M. every night to maintain his tolerance (he won't chew them because he hates the taste), and no one needs to fear his next PB&J encounter. Andrew is now 16 and recently earned his driver's license, which means far less parental supervision of where he goes and what he eats. The peace of mind OIT brought has been "huge," says Pete. "We sleep better at night."

As exciting as that result was, we needed to know how to make it last. Were people permanently desensitized after the two-year study, or did they have to continue taking peanut to keep the allergy at bay? To find out, we randomized everyone on the treatment arm to either a daily dose of peanut protein (300 milligrams) or placebo. A year later, 37 percent of the participants who'd taken that maintenance dose were still allergy-free, compared to 13 percent on the placebo arm. They also had lower levels of IgE antibodies and other allergy indicators in their blood. Many of the people who completed this study continue to eat peanut every day: sometimes one is enough; others have several. Many people maintain their tolerance with a daily dose of Peanut M&M's—it's not always a problem to take your medicine. Ongoing research is continuing to identify the best program for desensitizing the immune system and the best way to maintain that result.

ADDING DRUGS TO THE PROGRAM

As OIT research has evolved, a central question has been whether adding medications to the mix would improve outcomes. Over the past two decades, research at pharmaceutical and academic laboratories has led to new drugs that target key aspects of the immune system. It's logical to think that combining these with immunotherapy would benefit people seeking to overcome their food allergy. But we needed clinical trials to know for sure.

We tested this theory in a small clinical trial that combined a drug called omalizumab with OIT to treat multiple food allergies. Omalizumab is a monoclonal antibody created to reduce sensitivity to allergens and prescribed as a treatment for asthma. It works by binding to IgE antibodies, stopping them from igniting the events that result in an allergic reaction. Donald Leung and colleagues had tried omalizumab to increase the amount of peanut protein that a peanut-allergic person could eat in a food challenge. We built upon this knowledge in a new study. Eleven children who had a history of strong reactions to milk (hives, vomiting, anaphylaxis) and high levels of IgE antibodies received a nine-week course of omalizumab. After that, they moved on to OIT, plus seven more weeks of omalizumab. On the first day of OIT, the participants escalated from a milk powder dose of 0.1 milligram to a dose of 1,000 milligrams. They continued with daily doses, increased every week for up to eleven weeks. Of the 10 patients who completed this treatment (one dropped out on the first day of OIT due to a strong allergic reaction), 9 reached the point of tolerating a 2,000-milligram dose of milk. After the study ended, 9 patients were able to tolerate a normal amount of milk in their diet, and another could tolerate half that amount.

The first of our phase 1 studies enrolled twenty-five people allergic to two to five of the following: milk, egg, peanut, tree nuts, grains, and sesame seed. They took omalizumab for eight weeks and then added an OIT regimen customized to their set of allergies. The two treatments overlapped for eight weeks, and the study finished with eight weeks of OIT on its own. Although the participants did sometimes have allergic reactions to the treatment, nearly all were mild or moderate; only one required epinephrine. This study also showed us that omalizumab can speed up the time it takes for OIT to work. That's extremely promising, not only because the sooner a person is freed from allergies the better, but also because a faster program could be less expensive (we'll address cost concerns in the next chapter). Our second phase 1 study, which did not use omalizumab and lasted longer than the first, also proved safe.

SUMMARY OF SEVERAL KEY STUDIES OF ORAL IMMUNOTHERAPY (OIT) FOR PEANUT ALLERGY

FOCUS	STUDY DESIGN	NUMBER OF PARTICIPANTS	OUTCOMES	REFERENCE
Peanut OIT	A single-group study of OIT alone.	28	Twenty patients completed the study. Allergic symptoms were most common during the early part of the study, when the dose was first escalated. Patients rarely had allergic reactions when they took their doses at home.	Hofmann AM, et al. *J Allergy Clin Immunol*, 2009.
Peanut OIT	A single-group study of OIT alone.	29	Twenty-seven patients could safely eat 3.9 g of peanut in the oral food challenge at the end of the eight-month study.	Jones SM, et al. *J Allergy Clin Immunol*, 2009.

FOCUS	STUDY DESIGN	NUMBER OF PARTICIPANTS	OUTCOMES	REFERENCE
Peanut OIT	Randomized study comparing OIT with placebo.	19 for the OIT arm and 9 for the placebo arm	Three patients on the OIT arm left the study early because of allergic side effects. Of the remaining 16, all were able to consume 5,000 mg of peanut flour (about 20 peanuts) after a year of treatment, versus an average of 280 mg for the placebo patients.	Varshney P, et al. *J Allergy Clin Immunol*, 2011.
Peanut OIT	A single-group study of high-dose OIT.	22	After six weeks, 12 of 22 patients could eat 2.6 g of peanut protein. After thirty weeks, 16 patients could eat 6.6 g of peanut protein.	Anagnostou K, et al. *Clin Exp Allergy*, 2011.
Peanut OIT plus omalizumab	A single-group study combining omalizumab with OIT.	13	Twelve patients consumed 8,000 mg of peanut flour in an oral food challenge at the end of the study, up to 400 times what they could tolerate at the start. Two participants had severe reactions requiring treatment.	Schneider L, et al. *J Allergy Clin Immunol*, 2013.
Peanut OIT	A single-group study of OIT.	39	Twenty-four patients completed the study. Twelve patients completed an oral food challenge with 5,000 mg of peanut powder a month after the study finished, indicating that desensitization remained even after OIT was done.	Vickery BP, et al. *J Allergy Clin Immunol*, 2014.

FOCUS	STUDY DESIGN	NUMBER OF PARTICIPANTS	OUTCOMES	REFERENCE
Peanut OIT	A randomized study comparing OIT versus peanut avoidance. The latter group was allowed to switch to OIT after six months.	First phase: 39 on the OIT arm and 46 for the avoidance arm. Second phase: 45 from the avoidance arm underwent OIT	After six months, 24 of the 39 OIT recipients could safely consume 1,400 mg of peanut protein, compared with 0 of the 46 control patients. In the second phase, 24 of 45 patients who crossed over to the OIT arm could tolerate 1,400 mg of peanut protein. For 26 weeks after finishing treatment, nearly all patients could ingest 800 mg of peanut protein.	Anagnostou K, et al. *Lancet*, 2014.
Peanut OIT plus probiotic	A randomized, double-blind study comparing peanut OIT plus probiotic (*Lactobacillus rhamnosus*) with a placebo.	31 in each arm	Twenty-eight of the 31 patients on the treatment arm completed the therapy. Of those 28, 23 achieved sustained unresponsiveness (no allergic reaction, even after treatment finished) to 4,000 mg of peanut protein, versus 1 patient from the placebo arm.	Tang ML, et al. *J Allergy Clin Immunol*, 2015.

FOCUS	STUDY DESIGN	NUMBER OF PARTICIPANTS	OUTCOMES	REFERENCE
Peanut OIT plus omalizumab	Patients were randomized to receive either omalizumab or placebo, and then all patients underwent OIT.	29 on the omalizumab-plus-OIT arm and 8 on the placebo-plus-OIT arm	At the start of OIT, patients treated with omalizumab could tolerate up to 250 mg of peanut protein, versus 22.5 mg for patients given the placebo. After the OIT, 23 patients on the omalizumab-plus-OIT arm could tolerate 4,000 mg of peanut protein, compared to 1 patient on the placebo-plus-OIT arm.	MacGinnitie AJ, et al. *J Allergy Clin Immunol*, 2017.
Peanut OIT for very young children, ages 9 to 36 months	Children who tested positive for peanut allergy were blind-randomized to receive low-dose OIT (up to 300 mg) or high-dose OIT (up to 3,000 mg).	37 children total were enrolled; 20 received low-dose OIT and 17 received high-dose OIT.	Twenty-nine patients achieved sustained unresponsiveness (tolerance maintained four weeks after the study ended) to 5 g of peanut protein in an oral food challenge at the end of the study, including 17 of the 20 patients who received low-dose OIT and 12 of the 17 who received high-dose OIT.	Vickery BP, et al. *J Allergy Clin Immunol*, 2017.
Peanut OIT for moderate to severe allergy among children ages 6 to 18 years	A double-blind, randomized study of OIT versus placebo.	39 patients received OIT and 21 received a placebo.	Twenty-six of the 39 OIT patients tolerated 5 g of peanut protein at the oral food challenge when the study was done, compared to none of the placebo patients.	Kukkonen AK, et al. *Acta Paediatr*, 2017.

FOCUS	STUDY DESIGN	NUMBER OF PARTICIPANTS	OUTCOMES	REFERENCE
A follow-up of a peanut OIT plus probiotic study	Patients who completed a study of peanut OIT plus probiotic were assessed for allergen tolerance four years later.	In the original study, 24 underwent peanut OIT and 24 were given a placebo. Four years later, 12 OIT and 15 placebo patients underwent a double-blinded oral food challenge.	Four years after the original study, 16 of the 24 OIT patients were still eating peanut, compared to 1 of the 24 placebo patients. Among the 12 OIT patients who underwent the food challenge four years later, 7 had achieved sustained unresponsiveness to 4 g of peanut protein, versus 0 of the 15 placebo patients.	Hsiao KC, et al. *Lancet Child Adolesc Health,* 2017.
OIT with Palforzia (AR101) for peanut allergy	A randomized, double-blind trial of peanut OIT versus placebo.	29 patients received Palforzia (AR101) and 26 received the placebo.	Twenty-three of the 29 OIT patients tolerated 443 mg of peanut protein (compared to 5 of the 26 placebo patients) and 18 tolerated 1,043 mg of peanut protein (compared to 0 of the placebo patients) at the end of the study.	Bird JA, et al. *J Allergy Clin Immunol Pract,* 2018.
Peanut OIT for Japanese children	A single-group study of peanut OIT, using placebo data from a previous study as a comparison.	22 patients underwent peanut OIT. The historical control group included 11 patients.	Two years after completing OIT, 15 of the 22 patients could still tolerate 795 mg of peanut protein. Only 2 members of the historical control group completed their oral food challenge.	Nakagura K, et al. *Int Arch Allergy Immunol,* 2018.

FOCUS	STUDY DESIGN	NUMBER OF PARTICIPANTS	OUTCOMES	REFERENCE
Low-dose peanut OIT for children ages 3 to 17 years	A randomized study comparing peanut OIT maintained at 125 mg or 250 mg versus placebo.	31 children received OIT and 31 received the placebo.	Twenty-three of the 31 children treated with OIT tolerated at least 300 mg of peanut protein at a final oral food challenge, versus 5 of the 31 placebo patients. Thirteen of 31 OIT patients and 1 placebo patient tolerated 4.5 g of peanut protein at the final challenge.	Blumchen K, et al. *J Allergy Clin Immunol*, 2019.
OIT AR101 (Palforzia)	A large, randomized, phase 3 study comparing OIT with placebo.	551 people were enrolled. Of the 496 between the ages of 4 and 17 years, 372 received OIT and 124 received the placebo.	Of the 372 4- to 17-year-olds treated with OIT, 250 tolerated 600 mg or more of peanut protein at the final oral food challenge, versus 5 of the 124 adolescent participants who received the placebo. This clinical trial, known as PALISADE, was a landmark study toward the FDA approval of AR101.	Vickery BP, et al. *N Engl J Med*, 2018.

FOCUS	STUDY DESIGN	NUMBER OF PARTICIPANTS	OUTCOMES	REFERENCE
Peanut OIT	A randomized study comparing peanut OIT with an oat flour placebo.	60 patients were randomized to receive OIT up to 4,000 mg at 104 weeks and then avoidance (group 1); 35 patients were randomized to receive OIT up to 4,000 mg followed by 300 mg daily (group 2); and 25 were randomized to the placebo (group 3).	At week 104, 4,000 mg of peanut protein was safely tolerated by 51 of the 60 patients in group 1, 29 of the 35 patients in group 2, and 1 of the 25 placebo patients. At week 117, 21 of the 60 patients in group 1 could still tolerate 4,000 mg, after 13 weeks without consuming any peanut. In group 2, 19 of 35 patients tolerated 4,000 mg at week 117. At week 156, the end of the study, 8 of the 60 group 1 patients still tolerated 4,000 mg, as did 13 of the 35 group 2 patients.	Chinthrajah RS, et al. *Lancet,* 2019.

Tessa, whose story began this chapter, was among the participants in this first multi-allergy study. Her mother, Kim, had become desperate for help after the noodle-swapping episode brought Tessa to the brink of death. Tessa suffered emotionally, too. She'd been promoted to a competitive diving team but quit the sport due to anxiety over her food allergies. Kim recalls bringing her daughter to the house of a friend who'd invited her over for a pizza-making party. The kitchen was covered with flour when they arrived. "Mom," Tessa said as she took in the scene, "I can't be here."

Kim remembers how scared her daughter, then 9 years old, was at the beginning of the study. Here she was, a food-allergic child who'd ended up in the hospital on several occasions, deliberately exposing herself to her greatest enemies—all of them, all at once. Oral food challenges for the study lasted an entire summer. By December, she was ready to begin OIT. By May, she'd reached the maintenance doses for all her allergens. She could drink half a cup of milk. She could eat a piece of toast. "It was completely life-altering," says Kim. A *New York Times Magazine* story on OIT chronicled Tessa's transformation, including her first taste of cake and ice cream at the celebration commemorating the end of her study. Today Tessa can freely eat all of the foods that once threatened her life. She sleeps over at friends' houses and gets ice cream with them. Although it's taken time to overcome her anxiety, she is learning to rely on her body and trust the treatment that changed her life.

The results of studies like this involving omalizumab raised a crucial question: What difference did this drug make, exactly? We needed to compare OIT with and without omalizumab in a single study in order to be sure that adding it was truly beneficial. In a phase 2 study at Stanford, we randomized 48 children, ages 4 to 15 years, allergic to multiple foods to receive either OIT plus omalizumab or OIT plus a placebo. We also enrolled an additional 12 children as controls; they received no treatment at all. After 36 weeks, 30 of the 36 (83 percent) OIT-plus-omalizumab patients could tolerate 2 grams of protein containing the allergens they'd just been treated for, compared to 4 of the 12 OIT-plus-placebo patients (33 percent). The untreated group showed no meaningful changes in tolerance. Omalizumab, it seemed, could indeed make a difference.

SUMMARY OF KEY RANDOMIZED TRIALS OF IMMUNOTHERAPY FOR FOOD ALLERGIES OTHER THAN PEANUT

FOCUS	STUDY DESIGN	NUMBER OF PARTICIPANTS	OUTCOMES	REFERENCE
Oral immunotherapy (OIT) plus omalizumab for two to five allergies	This study had two stages. In the first part, all participants (ages 5–22 years) received omalizumab for 16 weeks plus OIT for all their allergens during weeks 8 to 30. Participants who could ingest at least 1 g of each of their allergens by weeks 28–29 were then blind-randomized to six weeks of 1 g of each allergen, 300 mg of each allergen, or no further exposure.	70 patients in the first stage, followed by 19 on the 1 g arm, 21 on the 300 mg arm, and 20 to discontinuation.	In an oral food challenge at the end of the study (week 36), 34 of the 40 patients on the two treatment arms could tolerate at least 2 g of each of their allergens, compared to 11 of the 20 patients on the discontinuation arm. The results suggest that continued exposure is best for staying desensitized.	Andorf S, et al. *Lancet,* 2019.
Epicutaneous immunotherapy (EPIT, or patch) for milk allergy in children	Patients were blind-randomized to receive either EPIT with milk powder or placebo.	18 children, ages 3 months to 15 years	EPIT was well tolerated by the treatment group. Children enrolled on the EPIT arm could tolerate a dose of 23.61 mg of milk by day 90, versus 1.77 mg at the start of the study.	Dupont C, et al. *J Allergy Clin Immunol,* 2010.

FOCUS	STUDY DESIGN	NUMBER OF PARTICIPANTS	OUTCOMES	REFERENCE
Long-term follow-up of OIT for egg allergy	Children (ages 5 to 18 years) with egg allergy received OIT for up to four years or placebo for one year or less.	55 patients total; 40 received OIT and 15 received the placebo.	By year 4, 20 of the 40 OIT patients showed sustained unresponsiveness to egg. None of the placebo patients passed the oral food challenge they were given at month 22.	Jones S, et al. *J Allergy Clin Immunol*, 2016.
OIT for wheat	Patients were randomized to either OIT with vital wheat gluten or placebo for one year. Those who passed the oral food challenge at that time continued for another year. Placebo patients could cross over to the treatment arm after the initial stage.	46 patients total, 23 on each arm	After a year of treatment, 12 of the 23 OIT patients and 0 of the placebo patients could tolerate at least 4,400 mg of wheat protein. At year 2, 7 of the 23 OIT patients could consume more than 7,400 mg of wheat protein. A food challenge given after avoiding wheat for eight to ten weeks following treatment showed that 3 OIT patients had achieved sustained unresponsiveness. Among the 21 placebo patients who crossed over to OIT after a year, 12 were desensitized to wheat after a year of treatment.	Nowak-Wegrzyn A, et al. *J Allergy Clin Immunol*, 2019.

DOES IMMUNOTHERAPY MAKE LIFE BETTER?

There's no use undergoing IT if it doesn't improve your life. That's the whole point of the program, and the promise of this new time for food allergy. But we can't assume that just because a treatment "works" that it's making people's lives better.

Numerous studies have confirmed that people with food allergy who go through OIT come out on the other side with greater well-being. In a study from Israel published in 2019, parents of 191 children, ages 4 to 12, who underwent OIT reflected on how the treatment changed their quality of life. Many of the parents reported an initial dip in quality of life when the study began—this stage can be difficult because it involves intentional allergic reactions. But by the time the children reached the maintenance dose, their lives were improved emotionally and socially.

A team of researchers in the UK measured quality of life as part of their 99-person (ages 7 to 15) randomized study of OIT for children with peanut allergy. Parents of participants who were 12 or younger completed a questionnaire specifically designed for gauging the well-being of children with food allergy. According to their responses, quality of life improved for all of the children on the study, and slightly more among those who underwent OIT. And other studies have shown that the treatment works for children and adults; no data so far show that younger patients have fared better on these studies than older patients.

Treating more than one food allergen at a time may improve quality of life even more. Multi-allergen immunotherapy studies around the world have demonstrated that a person can be desensitized to all their food allergens, a result that leads to meaningful changes for both the individual as well as their family and friends.

And what about the caregivers? Families with food-allergic children know very well that the grown-ups carry a burden of stress and anxiety about accidental exposure. Our team at Stanford asked more than 40 parents of children enrolled in an OIT study about whether the treatment improved their quality of life. Did their child's improved tolerance affect the choices they made for their family, such as social activities and restaurants? Did IT reduce the amount of time they spent preparing meals? Were they taking fewer precautions? Were they less anxious about their child's food allergy? The responses were illuminating. The burden shouldered by parents decreased significantly once their children were desensitized through IT. Questionnaires completed by parents of children on the placebo arm of the study did not show that change. Several more studies have shown a similar trend.

Life after immunotherapy isn't entirely carefree. We always recommend that people continue to carry allergy medication, including epinephrine, with them at all times, and remain vigilant, because unexpected allergic reactions can occur after consuming their daily small maintenance "dose" of peanut or other food. And it's best to help your immune system stay desensitized by continuing to eat at least one nut per day (every other day is also fine, but daily is better). The evidence suggests that OIT typically needs to continue for a long time. We do have data showing that desensitization remained in former peanut OIT patients who didn't eat nuts for a full year, but research is ongoing to test the long-term permanence of the treatment.

In later chapters, we'll look more closely at the psychological impact of food allergy. Understanding the emotional burden carried by children with food allergy, their families, and newly diagnosed adults is vastly important, and something the healthcare community has often underappreciated in the past. For the purposes of this OIT discussion, we have substantial evidence that the reduction in stress and anxiety and the release of restrictions that result from the treatment are deeply meaningful to food allergy families.

KEY STUDIES ON HOW OIT AFFECTS THE QUALITY OF LIFE OF PEOPLE WITH FOOD ALLERGIES AND THEIR FAMILIES

FOCUS	STUDY DESIGN	OUTCOMES	REFERENCE
OIT for children with milk allergy	30 children (ages 3 to 12 years) were treated. Their parents completed quality-of-life questionnaires before treatment and two months after finishing treatment.	OIT had a positive emotional impact, reduced food-related anxiety, and reduced social and dietary limitations for children and their families.	Carraro S, et al. *Int J Immunopathol Pharmacol*, 2012.
Caregivers with food-allergic children after OIT. Allergens included peanut, walnut, cashew, pecan, milk, egg, sesame, almond, and hazelnut.	Parents of children enrolled in two different clinical trials (OIT alone and OIT plus omalizumab) completed health-related quality-of-life questionnaires tailored to food allergies. A control group of parents whose children did not receive OIT was also included.	Parents of children in both studies (40 total) reported improvements in quality of life after treatment. The control group experienced no such significant changes.	Otani IM, et al. *Allergy Asthma Clin Immunol*, 2014.
OIT for children with peanut allergy	39 children (ages 7 to 16 years) were randomized to peanut OIT or peanut avoidance. The avoidance group could cross over to OIT after six months. Parents of participants ages 7 to 12 completed a food allergy quality-of-life questionnaire at the start and end of the study.	The quality-of-life scores were similar between the OIT and avoidance group at the start of the study. Both reported improvements, though these were slightly better for the treatment group.	Anagnostou K, et al. *Lancet*, 2014.

FOCUS	STUDY DESIGN	OUTCOMES	REFERENCE
Food-allergic patients during and after OIT. Allergens included milk, peanut, egg, sesame, and tree nuts.	A Food Allergy Quality of Life Questionnaire was given to parents of 191 children, ages 2 to 12, undergoing OIT for food allergy, at four times during and after treatment.	The questionnaire scores notably improved between the start of the study and reaching the maintenance dose. The worse the quality of life was at the start of the study, the more it improved by the end.	Epstein-Rigbi N, et al. *J Allergy Clin Immunol Pract,* 2019.
Peanut allergy with OIT plus probiotic	51 people randomized to either treatment (24) or placebo (27) from a larger trial completed the Food Allergy Quality of Life Questionnaire and the Food Allergy Independent Measure before, during, and after treatment.	Patients on the treatment arm reported significant improvements in their quality of life at three months after treatment and even more at twelve months after. Patients noted that it was their sustained unresponsiveness that accounted for the positive changes.	DunnGalvin A, et al. *Allergy,* 2018.
Low-dose peanut OIT	62 children, ages 3 to 17 years, were randomized to peanut OIT with a low (125 mg) or high (250 mg) maintenance dose or placebo. Changes in quality of life were measured through parental questionnaires.	The study authors reported a significant improvement in quality of life among patients randomized to the treatment arms.	Blumchen K, et al. *J Allergy Clin Immunol Pract,* 2019.

FOCUS	STUDY DESIGN	OUTCOMES	REFERENCE
Children undergoing peanut OIT and their parents	57 children were openly randomized to OIT and 20 to observation, and a Pediatric Quality of Life Inventory was completed by parents and children three times—before treatment, after one year, and after two years.	Thirty-seven children completed the entire study. Quality of life improved more among parents of treatment-group patients compared to parents of the observation-group patients. The children did not report the same improvements, raising the possibility that parents may have overestimated how OIT changed their children's lives.	Reier-Nilson T, et al. *Pediatr Allergy Immunol,* 2019.

OTHER TYPES OF IMMUNE THERAPY
Sublingual Immunotherapy

Although most immune therapy studies for food allergy have focused on the OIT route described so far, there are other methods. In the early 2000s, a group in Spain conducted the first study of sublingual immunotherapy (SLIT), in which small doses of the allergen are given as drops under the tongue. Researchers believe SLIT works by activating immune cells underneath the tongue, sending signals down the allergy pathway that curtail the response. The patient holds the drops there for a couple of seconds before swallowing. The study focused on hazelnut, a common allergen in children allergic to tree nuts and one that appears frequently in packaged foods such as pastries and ice creams. The researchers randomized 23 patients to hazelnut immunotherapy or placebo. By the end of the study, which lasted up to three months, participants on the treatment arm could tolerate far more hazelnut than patients on the placebo arm.

More studies followed. The NIH-funded Consortium of Food Allergy Research (CoFAR) conducted a double-blind, randomized trial of 40 peanut-allergic people, ages 12 to 37, comparing daily SLIT to placebo. In their 2013 report of the study, the researchers noted that a year of SLIT modestly desensitized most of the patients receiving the treatment. The researchers, led by David Fleischer in Denver, followed up on their initial report two years later, noting that three years after starting SLIT, the treatment had proven both effective at reducing the severity of peanut allergy for most patients and extremely safe, although they acknowledged that most patients hadn't kept up the treatment for the full three years.

Researchers at Johns Hopkins compared SLIT and OIT in a randomized study of 16 patients to see if one approach was better or safer. They concluded that OIT was more effective for treating peanut allergy but it also caused more side effects (allergic reactions), which made OIT studies harder for patients to stick with. Researchers from North Carolina looked at the long-term benefit of SLIT by giving the treatment to children with peanut allergy for up to five years. Of the 48 patients on the study, 32 could consume 750 milligrams of peanut protein at the end of the study, and 12 could consume 5,000 milligrams. Ten patients reached the level of sustained unresponsiveness. We are eagerly awaiting the results of ongoing SLIT studies.

Epicutaneous Immunotherapy

Then there's epicutaneous immunotherapy, or EPIT. This approach delivers allergen doses through a patch attached to the skin and works through a different immune system mechanism from oral routes. Essentially, a person wears their food allergen instead of eating it. Studies show that EPIT works by provoking the immune cells hiding underneath hair follicles, which in turn send signals that diminish the allergy response. A phase 1 study of 100 peanut-allergic people, ages 6 to 50, randomized to treatment with an allergen-delivering patch versus a placebo patch found that the experimental treatment was indeed safe. Some participants did have reactions, but the vast majority of these were mild or moderate. The patch, called Viaskin, appeared to warrant further investigation.

A phase 3 study soon followed. Researchers at several centers across the country, including Stanford, enrolled a total of 74 people, ages 4 to 25, with peanut allergy into a double-blind, randomized study comparing two different doses of the Viaskin Peanut patch (100 micrograms or 250 micrograms) and a placebo. The partici-pants took their doses for a full year, not knowing if they were re-ceiving the treatment or the placebo. If they could eat 5,044 mg of peanut protein at the end of the study, or at least ten times more than they could at the start, then their treatment was considered a success. Three of the 25 placebo patients reached that goal. So did 11 of the 24 patients with the low-dose patch and 12 of the 25 patients with the high-dose patch. Children under 11 fared best of all. The EPIT-treated patients had higher levels of IgG4 and lower levels of IgE—both indicators of a retrained immune system—at the end of the study. Side effects were common but minor; no patients were in danger from allergic reactions to the patch.

Leah Cuellar, the parent who decided to keep peanuts in the house, as we wrote about in chapter 4, enrolled her son, William, in this study at Stanford. William was 2½ years old when he started. The oral food challenge at the start of the study was tough. He turned red and vomited after eating about two peanuts' worth of peanut protein over three hours. But Leah was determined, even though she wasn't sure if her son was receiving the patch that con-tained peanut protein. She knew how much it would mean for him to live without having to fear peanuts. It was hard to keep a toddler from pulling off the patch. "He wore a lot of onesies," she recalls. Because William was already coping with the patch and the trial, Leah and her husband, Hector, decided to delay potty training for a little while. After the initial study, William continued with the treatment, now definitively receiving the patch containing peanut protein. He remained on the treatment for three years. Although he's too young to say, his parents wholeheartedly believe the time and effort were worthwhile to make him safe from allergic reactions to peanuts.

And because the treatment requires very little of the participants—they don't have to remember to take their peanut powder at home; they don't have to worry about travel plans disrupting their dose routine; children don't have to eat a food that they don't like— nearly all of the participants stuck with the regimen for the full year. The patch approach is also being studied for allergies to milk and other foods. The FDA is currently reviewing the patch for approval, potentially adding to what we hope will one day be a long list of therapies to choose from.

Probiotics and Immunotherapy

There's one more spoke on the immunotherapy wheel: adding a probiotic. Because research has suggested close ties between the gut microbiome and the immune system, it's reasonable to wonder whether adding healthy gut flora to OIT could enhance the benefit. Researchers in North Carolina and Australia joined forces to see if combining peanut OIT with doses of bacteria called *Lactobacillus rhamnosus* could bring children with peanut allergy to sustained unresponsiveness. That "Holy Grail" of treatment results had yet to be attained when the study began, and the researchers hoped that adding a probiotic to OIT would tip the scales. According to their 2015 report, among the 28 participants randomized to the treatment arm (OIT plus probiotic), 23 had no allergic reaction to peanut up to five weeks after the study finished. Among the 28 randomized to the placebo arm, just 1 patient had that outcome. Not enough time had elapsed to know whether the tolerance remained, but the results were certainly intriguing. Four years later, the researchers reported that the benefit from the combination of OIT and probiotic had lasted.

Probiotic research is tricky, but immunologists are continuing to explore the use of healthy gut flora as part of the quest to restore the immune system to its nonallergic state.

WHAT THE MEDICAL AUTHORITIES SAY ABOUT IMMUNOTHERAPY

All the data researchers have amassed on IT for food allergy prompted leading medical organizations to weigh in. In 2017, the European Academy of Allergy and Clinical Immunology (EAACI) released an extensive review of the research and recommendations concerning the use of immunotherapy to treat food allergy. The agency's current suggestions are phrased cautiously. According to a review of the data, the guidelines note that strong evidence favors the use of OIT to increase tolerance to milk in children who are enrolled in OIT studies. Because ideal treatment regimens are still being worked out, and long-term data on the duration of desensitization are not yet available, the EAACI said the evidence so far did not support recommending OIT as a program to reverse food allergy. However, the agency did acknowledge that at least one randomized controlled trial accomplished exactly that. The guidelines were the same for egg OIT, although the agency noted that the one randomized trial found that half of the participants had "sustained unresponsiveness"—that is, continued desensitization after finishing the treatment. For peanut OIT at this point, the agency recommends it for desensitization only in the context of clinical trials. For the patch approach and the under-the-tongue method, the reviewers concluded that more studies are needed.

Although these suggestions seem tentative, they are encouraging. We are still in the early days of this new era, and health authorities must always exercise extreme caution because so many medical professionals and patients depend on their guidance. The fact that these guidelines exist is a huge breakthrough in itself. And the agency has embraced OIT to the extent it deems possible given the research so far. The guidelines also emphasize that OIT must be conducted by a medical professional at a medical facility. In 2019, the Australasian Society of Clinical Immunology and Allergy (ASCIA) advised that OIT remain solely within the context of clinical trials until more studies are completed and the treatment is standardized.

The American Academy of Pediatrics has gone one step further. "Under close medical supervision," the organization wrote in May 2019, "peanut OIT can be safe and effective for raising the threshold of allergen needed to trigger an allergic reaction for many patients." In other words, OIT can improve tolerance for people with peanut allergy. The approach, the recommendation continued, "may potentially decrease the risk for severe allergic reactions due to accidental or unintentional allergen exposures."

As this short announcement from the AAP also noted, researchers haven't come to a consensus on the best immunotherapy regimen for any food allergy, whether single or multiple. That's where the dozens of ongoing studies come in. "It is likely that the food allergy treatment landscape will look very different in 10 years," the AAP concluded. We agree entirely. And it's the people living with food allergy today—readers of this book, study participants, and families who courageously step into this new landscape—who are making that very different-looking future a reality.

FOOD ALLERGY VACCINES

We have one stop before ending this survey of the territory traveled by the research so far. One of the most common questions we hear about food allergy is whether a vaccine is possible. In this setting, the word *vaccine* doesn't mean inoculating a person against a disease by exposing them to small amounts of it, as is the case with polio, measles, and the like. Food allergies are not infections. Food allergy vaccines are more akin to the vaccines being developed for cancer treatment. They work on people already diagnosed with food allergy by resetting the immune system. Patients receive an injection of DNA encoding a particular food protein, which is then absorbed into cells. The presence of this new DNA in the body disrupts the usual response the body takes against that food protein. The approach, also known as peptide immunotherapy, avoids the daily-dose requirements of other immunotherapies. A food allergy vaccine also avoids the necessity of eating the allergen, something many people fear at the outset.

In a phase 1 study of a peanut vaccine called PVX108, 6 people underwent increasing doses of either the vaccine or a placebo. Afterward, another 18 participants received six injections of the highest dose over sixteen weeks. The treatment was safe, eliciting side effects that were easily manageable. Another study confirmed that the vaccine did not trigger allergic reactions—a logical concern, since the vaccine contains peanut protein—by examining blood samples from 146 peanut-allergic donors. Basophil cells, which become activated during an allergic reaction, did not become activated in the presence of PVX108. Another peanut vaccine, HAL-MPE1, has also survived a phase 1 study. Although the results weren't as strong as the PVX108 study, the experimental treatment was safe and is continuing its walk on the clinical trial path.

A later chapter on the not-so-distant future of food allergy includes more about vaccines—particularly one known as LAMP DNA that we are following eagerly.

IMMUNOTHERAPY: WHAT WE KNOW SO FAR

TYPE OF THERAPY	WHAT THE STUDIES HAVE SHOWN
ORAL IMMUNOTHERAPY (OIT)	
Stand-alone therapy (food "dose" only, no additional medications)	• OIT has desensitized study participants with allergies to peanut, milk, egg, and other foods. • Many patients experienced mild side effects, although severe reactions can occur. • Desensitization was often temporary. After the study ended, the food allergy sometimes returned. • Studies of peanut powder showed high rates of desensitization and side effects.
OIT with omalizumab	• When patients were given omalizumab before and during OIT, they became desensitized to their allergen(s) within weeks, instead of the months or years seen with stand-alone OIT. • Including omalizumab improved the safety of OIT. • Omalizumab plus OIT has desensitized study participants to multiple allergens at once. • A drawback to omalizumab treatment is the high cost of the medication.
OIT with probiotics	• In a randomized study, participants remained desensitized to their allergen even four years after treatment finished, longer than patients given a placebo. • This study did not include an OIT-alone treatment arm, making the benefit of the probiotic difficult to interpret.

TYPE OF THERAPY	WHAT THE STUDIES HAVE SHOWN
OIT with FAHF-2 (traditional Chinese herbal blend)	• Studies of this approach have had mixed results. • A phase 2 study of OIT in combination with omalizumab and FAHF-2 for the treatment of multiple food allergens is currently under way. • Scientists do not yet fully understand how FAHF-2 might work as a food allergy treatment.
OIT with dupilumab	• Dupilumab is an anti-IL-4R antibody currently approved for the treatment of eczema and asthma. • Studies of this drug in combination with OIT or as an addition to OIT plus peanut powder are under way. • The benefit of dupilumab in the treatment of food allergy is still to be determined.
SUBCUTANEOUS IMMUNOTHERAPY (SCIT)	
Stand-alone therapy	• Initial studies found SCIT to be effective for treating peanut allergy. • However, the high rates of severe side effects made this approach unacceptable.
SCIT using aluminum hydroxide	• Some research suggests that adding aluminum hydroxide to SCIT may decrease the immune system's response to an allergen. • A phase 1 study of HAL-MPE1 (a peanut extract that enters the body adhered to aluminum) found this agent to be safe. • A phase 2 trial is currently under way for mCyp c1, a modified version of a protein tied to fish allergy, suspended in aluminum.
SUBLINGUAL IMMUNOTHERAPY (SLIT)	
Stand-alone therapy	• Clinical trials of SLIT for kiwi, peanut, milk, hazelnut, and peach have been completed. • These studies show that SLIT is less effective than OIT but also causes fewer side effects.

TYPE OF THERAPY	WHAT THE STUDIES HAVE SHOWN
EPICUTANEOUS IMMUNOTHERAPY (EPIT)	
Skin patch	• Clinical trials of skin patches have been completed for the treatment of peanut and milk allergies. • A phase 3 study of Viaskin (a proprietary patch) for peanut allergy showed a benefit for this treatment, but the study did not meet additional requirements needed to confirm the treatment worked. • A clinical trial of this patch for the treatment of milk allergy is ongoing.
MONOCLONAL ANTIBODIES (STAND-ALONE THERAPY)	
Etokimab	• Etokimab is an antibody that acts against IL-33, an immune system cell that plays a role in food allergy. • Data from a phase 2 study suggested that this drug is safe and may desensitize people to peanut allergens in as little as one dose.
VACCINES	
EMP-123	• This vaccine includes three proteins commonly involved in peanut allergy (Ara h1, Ara h2, and Ara h3). • In a phase 1 study, patients experienced a high rate of side effects, sometimes severe.
PVX108	• This peanut vaccine includes synthetic versions of components of common peanut allergens. • Preliminary results from a phase 1 trial suggest that this vaccine is safe for the treatment of peanut allergy.
DNA LAMP vaccine (ASP0892)	• With this approach, patients receive an injection of the DNA encoding a protein allergen, rather than the protein itself. • A phase 1 study of this vaccine for the treatment of adults with peanut allergy is in progress.

This overview of the research so far is hardly exhaustive, but gives a clear map of IT country. And the question that you may now be asking is *Could this work for me? Could this work for my child?* That's where the next chapter comes in.

THE BOTTOM LINE

- Studies show that immunotherapy effectively desensitizes people with food allergy, though side effects sometimes occur.

- Immunotherapy retrains the immune system so that it no longer produces IgE, the antibodies responsible for triggering allergic symptoms.

- The most common immunotherapy is oral. But sublingual (under the tongue) and epicutaneous (through the skin) approaches are also being tested in clinical trials.

- This field of research is burgeoning, with biologic drugs (such as monoclonal antibodies) and probiotics that can be added to immunotherapy or used on their own, vaccines, and other approaches currently under investigation.

- The first immunotherapy drug has now been approved for the treatment of peanut allergy.

Chapter 8

IMMUNOTHERAPY AND YOU

*How treatment works, where to find it,
and deciding if it's right for you*

On a vacation in Florida, Kim Hartman ran into some friends from New York at a restaurant. The couple's son was there, sitting with them at the table eating French fries like any other child might be. Kim burst into tears when she saw him.

The son suffered from food allergy. Kim knew his parents well enough to know that they did not bring him to restaurants. He did not order food off a menu like a regular customer. They never took risks like that. Yet here they were, and Kim had just one question: "How can I get my son to be like yours?"

In early 2017, two pediatric allergists at Johns Hopkins University set out to understand why people were pursuing OIT. The treatment wasn't fully embraced by the medical community, yet an increasing number of families were seeking it out through both clinical trials and private clinics. The researchers figured if they had a better grasp on what was motivating this trend, they could shape food allergy therapy accordingly.

They distributed a survey to families with children who had either gone through OIT or were in the midst of it. About 75 of the 123 respondents said the reason they sought OIT was to reduce the risk of a deadly allergic reaction. A dozen or so said their chief goal was "reducing the hassle of strict avoidance," and slightly fewer said their main concern was adding the allergen into their child's routine diet. For most of them, success meant that although the child might still avoid the food, the allergic reaction would be less likely and also less severe. Many parents worried about fatal anaphylaxis. They had anxiety about their children dying. They found avoiding foods to be difficult. They wanted their children to try OIT because they wanted them to be safe.

That was certainly what Kim was after for her son, Andy. After his first allergic reaction—a birthday party when he was 13 months old ended with a trip to the nearest emergency room—Andy was diagnosed with allergy to peanut, egg, and all tree nuts. He was about 10 years old when Kim cried at the sight of her friends in Florida. With extraordinary perseverance, she found her way to our clinic at Stanford at the right time: the FDA had just given us permission to conduct a multi-allergy trial especially for patients with IgE levels that were too high for our other studies, a category that Andy fit into.

Andy and his mother traveled from New York to California every two weeks at first, missing days of eighth grade so his doses could be escalated. Over time their trips shifted to every other month. "He wanted this really badly," Kim recalls.

But the treatment wasn't always easy. Andy developed eosinophilic esophagitis (EoE), an allergic condition in which the esophagus becomes inflamed from white blood cells collecting in the tissue. It's a rare and treatable side effect of OIT that can cause abdominal pain and unpredictable vomiting. For Andy, that included a couple of occasions at school. Kim worried about what the treatment was putting him through not just physically but also emotionally. "That's embarrassing for an eighth-grade boy," says Kim.

OIT took a toll on Kim, too. She fielded criticism from friends and family telling her she was doing the wrong thing, especially when the EoE developed. She kept a brave face in front of her son, but privately she sometimes wondered why they were trying this pioneering therapy.

But then she would remember exactly why they were doing it. She would hear Andy's fear about going somewhere nuts might be present. She would make vacation plans that had to revolve around his allergy needs. She would worry about an accidental nut exposure when they were least expecting it. She would steel herself and set her hesitation to one side. "I always took the attitude that either you're in or you're out," she says. "Either we were going to trust in this approach, or we weren't going to get through it."

They got through it—and then some. Andy's commitment eventually enabled him to consume eight different types of nuts, including peanut. The EoE disappeared with continued oral immunotherapy. When he was a sophomore in high school, Andy traveled with his class to Peru, a trip he never would have made before OIT. He went away to college to pursue his love of theater, straying farther from home than he might have before. He doesn't feel the need to tell a restaurant server about his allergies anymore. And he really likes Nutella. "He lives a much different life than he would have if he hadn't done this," says Kim. So do his parents.

For many families, the decision to pursue OIT isn't made just once; it's made again and again. It's a commitment, and like any commitment, it's not always easy to maintain. The thousands of children and adults who are now free from the fear of severe allergic reactions have repeatedly strengthened our commitment and belief in the power of this program to reverse the condition. But families considering OIT for food allergy face a range of considerations. This chapter offers a guided tour through the world of OIT. The food allergy families Kari and her team worked with over the past decade plus have taught us so much about the sights and scenes—the challenges and the rewards. We hope this vast experience can now benefit those approaching the foothills.

Before we proceed, one more word. Food allergy families: We see you. We know how resilient and brave you are. We know the perils you face and the determination it takes to ensure the safety of your children and yourselves. And we know that much of what you go through is hidden—the stress, the fear, the frustration. And we want to assure you that this new era of food allergy is here to help. We can't guarantee a life free from stress or even free from the challenges of a confused immune system. But we can promise you that the future of food allergy is much different from its past—much better—and there's room for everyone.

WHO CAN DO IMMUNOTHERAPY?

In theory, anyone with food allergy can undergo immunotherapy. Starting immunotherapy at a very young age has advantages. Many children develop aversions to their allergen, partly because they've spent their whole life up to the time of treatment being warned away from that food and partly because the food hasn't been part of their diet. The younger children are, the less of a chance that they will put up a fuss about eating the food.

Yet a person is also never too old to start immunotherapy. Clinical trials have enrolled patients in their fifties, and some aspects of the treatment have no age limit. Because the process can elicit allergic reactions, it's important that participants be in good health. OIT is a retraining of the immune system, so it's important that this system isn't preoccupied with other serious illnesses.

Scott Jung was 29 when he decided to enroll in a clinical trial at Stanford. He'd grown up allergic to peanuts, tree nuts, and fish, but when an allergist tested him as an adult, he discovered his tree nut allergy had disappeared. The pistachios, almonds, Brazil nuts, and macadamias he'd avoided all his life now posed no threat. That change made Scott, who lives in the San Francisco Bay Area, wonder if there was any way he could get rid of his peanut allergy. His allergist pointed him toward our trials at Stanford and he enrolled in a peanut allergy vaccine study. "I got up to ten peanuts without a reaction," he recalls. "It was a significant improvement. It was amazing." Scott's tolerance was a short-lived benefit of the study and it wore off eventually. Motivated more by lifestyle than fear, he hopes to try immunotherapy in the near future. "I like foods that typically have peanuts in them," he says. "It would be worth it to give it a shot."

WILL IT HURT?

Anyone starting immunotherapy should be clear about what the treatment entails. In the bluntest terms: you are consuming a substance that your body believes is poisonous. We say this not to scare you but because we believe it's best to start this process clear-eyed about the road ahead.

Immunotherapy begins with an oral food challenge, which takes about four hours, to confirm the presence of an allergy. Many individuals with a food allergy diagnosis have never undergone this test. An egg allergy may have been diagnosed through a skin prick test after an allergic reaction to something else. Some people come to immunotherapy for tree nuts never having eaten a single tree nut. So the clinician (and the patient) need to be sure that the allergy actually exists.

The very purpose of an oral food challenge is to provoke a reaction. For this reason, the test is always conducted by a medical professional at a medical facility. Epinephrine is on hand. A crash cart is standing by in case of anaphylaxis. A supervised oral food challenge carries minuscule risk, but if the patient has the allergy in question, then a reaction will occur. That's the whole point of the test. Some patients find oral food challenges scary; some parents do, too. They are an unavoidable part of immunotherapy, but that doesn't mean they're easy. On the bright side, young patients usually appreciate the chance to watch movies, read, write, or draw during the time period following each new dose. "I watched *The Hunger Games* all day, ate nuts, and waited to have an allergic reaction," says Violet Barnett, Sloan's daughter, who began immunotherapy for tree nut allergies when she was in fifth grade. She became sick of the movie as she became un-sick from nuts.

Immunotherapy works similarly to an oral food challenge—the doses start small and increase slowly. However, oral food challenges are designed to elicit allergic reactions. In contrast, immunotherapy is designed to desensitize by increasing the doses in very small increments and over longer amounts of time. The purpose of an oral food challenge is to find your tolerance threshold. The purpose of immunotherapy is to get you well. As the previous chapter described, many immunotherapy studies begin by moving the patient rapidly to a "baseline" dose, which marks the starting point for the study. That baseline dose is often low enough not to trigger an allergic reaction. Again, that's the point. The goal of immunotherapy is to increase the amount of a food a person can tolerate before their body reacts. Some patients want to push that desensitization to the point of consuming the food freely—that is, to no longer have the allergy whatsoever. Others are content with increasing their tolerance enough so that severe reactions to accidental exposures are no longer a concern.

Melanie Thernstrom says she recently had the thrill of checking the "no allergies" box on a school form for her son, Kieran. "Food allergy is now a problem we don't have," she says. "We have just completely crossed it off our list." But that reward was hard-won. The process had been long. Kieran's treatment had taken two years. Although many children were taking omalizumab in combination with immunotherapy by the time Kieran began his treatment, he was too young for the drug. Omalizumab typically speeds up the allergen introduction process because it can block the immune system from reacting to the food protein. Patients who undergo oral immunotherapy with no accompanying drug often proceed more slowly because allergic reactions occur more frequently. "It was two steps forward and one step back," Melanie says of the process. Some days it seemed Kieran was becoming more used to an allergen. Other days he would break out in hives and his lips would swell, and his dose had to be reduced. "My food hurt me," Kieran would cry.

Yet Melanie says she always knew that whatever challenges OIT brought, it far surpassed the alternative. "It's hard," she says of OIT, "but living life with food allergies is miserable and I knew it would only get more miserable."

That doesn't mean immunotherapy with omalizumab is easy. The drug comes in the form of a thick liquid that must be injected, a treatment that isn't comfortable. For caregivers, all immunotherapy involves some degree of watching and waiting for a child to become sick from an allergen. There is no way around that reality, even as we work to make immunotherapy faster and more comfortable.

It's not easy to watch any child have an allergic reaction, let alone your own. At our clinic at Stanford, we try to make our pediatric patients as comfortable as possible. They're courageous and we want them to feel like the heroes that they are. We want children to leave their visits trusting that the hospital is a safe and caring place. We believe all pediatric allergists have the same attitude. Yes, there will be times when we need to give your children a little tough love so that they keep going with the increases in dose. But we do this because we know what lies on the other side: freedom.

HOW LONG DOES IT TAKE?

The simple, if unsatisfying, answer to this common question is that OIT takes as long as it takes. The duration depends in part on the goal. As Kim Yates, whom we wrote about in chapter 7, puts it, "There's the live-with-it camp and the fix-it camp." Some families are content with reaching the point where they no longer have to worry about a severe allergic reaction to a tiny amount of the food. Many people with food allergy can reach that point within six months of starting treatment. Others want the comfort of knowing that they can eat whatever they want, whenever they want, in whatever amount they want.

The ability to safely consume about 300 milligrams of an allergen (whether in the form of food flour or the food itself) typically means a person is safe from cross-contamination. Nut-free packaged foods made at facilities that process nuts are safe at this level of desensitization. At 1,000 milligrams, a person is considered "bite proof," meaning a bite of allergen does not awaken the sleeping immune system sentries. That level protects the young child who snags a cookie from the holiday treats table the moment you look away, or the well-meaning relative who insists that food allergy isn't real. Tolerating between 2,000 and 4,000 milligrams of an allergen typically means tolerating an entire serving.

Each of these levels requires a different duration of IT—the more desensitized a person wishes to become, the higher the quantity they need to tolerate, and thus the longer the treatment. Deciding about what level of desensitization to aim for can depend on several factors. Some people have such a high level of IgE antibodies that reaching the point where the allergy disappears completely may not be realistic. In such cases, it may seem pointless to push beyond 300 milligrams. As Stanford physician Tina Sindher puts it, we need to reach a level where accidental ingestion is safe before going to higher doses. Reaching a dose that makes a person safe from accidental exposure typically takes around six months. Full desensitization can take up to two years. Speeding up this time frame is one of the goals of immunotherapy research. The addition of omalizumab to OIT quickened the pace at which patients could tolerate their next higher dose, and we hope to get faster still. But the therapy is still new and patients differ from one another (a vital aspect of immunotherapy that we will cover in a later chapter). As the treatment evolves, we will have more clearly defined regimens and a host of options for patients to choose from.

HOW MUCH DOES IT COST?

As with any medical intervention, the cost of immunotherapy is a crucial consideration for many families and individuals. Healthcare expenses are formidable in the United States, amounting to an estimated $3.5 trillion per year, or about $10,379 per person. That's about 18 percent of the country's entire gross domestic product. It is unsafe to try immunotherapy without the supervision of a medical professional, but that means the treatment carries a price tag. Cost will inevitably weigh heavily into any family discussions about immunotherapy.

Immunotherapy isn't yet widely covered by insurance because the approach is still considered experimental. Typically, companies submit the evidence gathered in clinical trials to the FDA, which then reviews the data and approves (or rejects) the drug for marketing. Insurance companies determine their coverage offerings based on whether a particular intervention has gained approval by the FDA and whether the major medical authority in a particular field considers the intervention to be the standard treatment for the illness in question. Both of these milestones depend on data. Immunotherapy is just beginning to cross the chasm separating the experimental from the established.

AR101, a medication made of peanut powder, is the first product to reach the other side. Others, like EPIT, are close behind. These concrete advances legitimize the field of immunotherapy in the eyes of the insurance company executives who grant (or don't grant) coverage.

This state of affairs for immunotherapy has several implications where cost is concerned. For clinical trial participants, care is paid for by the grants that support the trial. The money for large clinical trials usually comes from a combination of federal research grants and pharmaceutical companies. The companies that provide support for a clinical trial typically have a stake in the research—namely, their product is part of the experimental treatment. That involvement raises the obvious concern about bias. If a company is providing funding for a trial testing its own product, then isn't the study more likely to show a favorable result? This concern is reasonable. But it's also important to understand that very few large clinical trials proceed without commercial support. Simply put, federal agencies do not have enough research dollars to support all the worthy work currently under way. Biotechnology companies and other manufacturers typically have funding that equals or surpasses the amount awarded through research grants. And these companies know that without clinical trials, their products will not become widely available.

That doesn't mean clinical trial participants have no expenses. Travel costs can be formidable. Immunotherapy is not widely available and studies tend to be concentrated at academic institutions with researchers dedicated to this particular field. Therefore individuals wishing to enroll in studies may have a substantial journey— physically, not just metaphorically—to reach a trial site. Our wish is for anyone who wants immunotherapy to have access to it, geographically and financially. Families have traveled to Stanford from across the country. But obviously making that trip depends on having the means to do so. Participating in an immunotherapy trial may also carry some medical costs if you or your child has allergic reactions following the daily dose of allergen taken at home. These short-term expenses may save money in the long run if immunotherapy eliminates the need for epinephrine and trips to the hospital. However, it may be helpful to factor in some amount of unpredictable expense.

The Schatz family, whose story was included in the last chapter, lives just fifteen minutes from their trial center, so travel costs were not an issue when Andrew, now 16, underwent immunotherapy. But his mother, Leilani, acknowledges that taking their son to his trial appointments required taking off from work, which can be a financial burden for some families. Overall, she says the cost was minimal, "especially given the peace of mind we gained from knowing that Andrew is less at risk of an accidental exposure."

Other families have dug deeper into their bank accounts. For Eric Graber-Lopez, whose son, Sebastian, we met in chapter 4, oral immunotherapy was a steep investment. They flew from Boston to Palo Alto every two weeks for about fifteen months so Sebastian could participate in a multi-food allergy trial at Stanford. The travel expenses totaled about $45,000. "It was not an insignificant expense," notes Eric. But he and his wife were fortunate to have the resources and believed the investment was well worth it. "It was a little nuts," he says, "but I think it's probably the best decision we ever made regarding his care." Obviously a travel expense like this puts clinical trials out of reach for many, if not most, families, even though studies themselves carry no cost. There are other options, however, which we'll come to soon.

As immunotherapy drugs gain FDA approval, we will learn more about their price tags. AR101 costs several thousand dollars for the first six months of treatment, and then several hundred dollars per month after that initial period. Insurance carriers will presumably cover most of this expense. The out-of-pocket amount should be much lower, although it's impossible to be certain and obviously it will vary depending on the insurance plan.

There are multiple ways to view drug costs. At a national level, economists consider how heavy a burden the price of a medication is on a country's healthcare system. How much will immunotherapy cost the country? The World Health Organization calculates whether a drug is worth the dollars through the lens of a country's gross domestic product. Wealthier countries can afford more expensive drugs than poorer countries (which is one reason why the same drug carries many different price tags around the world). According to the WHO's interpretation, a drug is cost effective—meaning, it's worth the price—in the United States if the expense per person comes to $50,000 per year or less.

The Institute for Clinical and Economic Review (ICER), an independent research organization that evaluates the economic value of medical interventions, takes a more detailed tack. ICER ranks beneficial drugs as high value if they cost less than $50,000 to $100,000 per quality-adjusted life year (a measure that takes into account both the quantity and quality of life). Those that cost between $101,000 and $150,000 but offer an important benefit are ranked as intermediate value, while those that exceed $150,000 are denoted as low value. An ICER report from June 2019 noted that AR101 would have to cost no more than $4,808 per year to achieve the highest rank of cost effectiveness ($100,000 per quality-adjusted life year). A cost of $7,248 per year would put AR101 at the high end of the intermediate category. Given these estimates, the Institute calculated that 41 percent of people who are eligible for AR101 could receive the treatment in a given year without taking a harmful toll on the country's healthcare system.

Then in the summer of 2019, ICER declared that the benefit of AR101 and the peanut patch were not worth the risk—nor, by implication, the cost. That position was flawed. As a large team of allergists noted in response, patients undergo immunotherapy aware of the side effects. As anyone with food allergy knows, it's the accidental exposure that is concerning, not the deliberate reaction induced for the purpose of improving tolerance. And as study after study has shown, people with food allergy and parents of children with the condition report that their lives improved after treatment. A study of epicutaneous peanut immunotherapy and oral peanut immunotherapy found that both approaches will likely be cost-effective. The more data we have from clinical trials, the more we will understand about how many cases of anaphylaxis these treatments ultimately prevent and how long patients remain desensitized.

In the short term, families participating in clinical trials need to consider travel expenses and any financial loss due to the necessary visits to the clinic for periodic dose increases. Conversely, cost deliberations can also include the money that will be saved from not having to go to the hospital for severe allergic reactions and the possibility of not filling prescriptions for epinephrine each year. Every family will weigh their pros and cons according to what works best for them. In the longer term, we believe that immunotherapy programs will become widely available and increasingly accessible. Picture a world in which everyone who wants to become desensitized to a food allergen can be—that's the world we are working toward.

WILL IMMUNOTHERAPY CURE MY FOOD ALLERGY?

As we wrote about above, the outcome of any immunotherapy treatment depends on a patient's goal. Do you want the ability to consume your former allergen with abandon? Do you dream of the moment Melanie Thernstrom described, of not having to list your child's food allergies on school and camp forms? Or are you content with knowing that an accidental bite won't cause your or your child's throat to close up? Do you want to eat ice cream without restrictions, or are you happy with knowing that a drop of milk spilled on your food won't cause harm? The answers to these questions influence the result of immunotherapy.

But it's also too soon to tell whether immunotherapy desensitizes a person for good. We don't have enough long-term data to know how long it lasts. It's impossible to know if patients remain unresponsive for ten years or more following a study completed just three years ago. Currently many patients continue with a maintenance dose of allergen following immunotherapy. For some people, like Andrew Schatz, maintenance means swallowing a single peanut every night. Other people consume many more than that. Axel Thomas completed a peanut desensitization study when he was almost 6 years old. He could tolerate up to 5,000 milligrams of peanut at that time, enough to keep him safe from a dangerous reaction. The trial required him to stop the treatment for seven months to see if his tolerance lasted. At his next food challenge, he ate 33 peanuts' worth of peanut butter. To keep that result, he eats two peanut M&M's every night. Axel's mother, Anne, remembers being told that her only option was to be afraid of nuts and to teach Axel to feel the same way. Maintaining his tolerance with a bit of nightly candy, says Anne, has been empowering.

Immunologists studying food allergy often refer to these differences as *tolerance* and *desensitization*. In the strict definition of tolerance, the immune system is unresponsive to the protein that once triggered an antibody attack. The cellular mechanisms that once made the body break out in hives, swell, and seize up in pain have disappeared, become dormant, or been suppressed. As a result, a formerly allergic person will not develop symptoms no matter how many peanuts or wheat or eggs they eat. This state is also sometimes referred to by the milder term, *sustained unresponsiveness*. This phrase, as jargonish as it may be, is perhaps the most accurate. We can't yet guarantee that an allergy is gone forever. Rather, we are actively watching how long tolerance lasts—how long unresponsiveness is sustained.

By contrast, some patients end up desensitized rather than tolerant. The term *desensitization* refers to a more temporary halt of the allergy that depends on continuing to expose the immune system to the culprit protein on a regular basis. Stop those two evening M&M's, and the allergy returns. Because we don't yet know enough about which regimens lead to tolerance or which patients are most likely to achieve that result, maintenance doses are frequently recommended after clinical trials. We want all the hard work of going through immunotherapy to pay off as richly as possible.

In studies completed so far, typically some percentage of patients end up tolerant to the allergen and some end up desensitized. Clinical trials have not managed to bring all patients into sustained unresponsiveness, but they certainly haven't left patients back where they started, either. The current regimens waver between desensitization and tolerance for those who complete them fully. And a major purpose of ongoing research is to increase the percentage of patients who become tolerant, their unresponsiveness sustained for the rest of their lives.

The goal of food allergy treatment research is to find a cure. We want everyone with food allergies to reach a state where they can freely eat the allergen without fear. But like so many other fields, allergy researchers rarely use the word *cure*.

Physicians hesitate to say that a food allergy is cured because we can't predict the future. It overpromises. *Cure* is inextricably tied to media hype followed by the public feeling let down. We have been barraged with sensational headlines of the next big thing in medicine, only to be disappointed when a treatment turns out to be less than optimal. Even if a clinical trial ended with all patients desensitized to their allergen for years and years, doctors would still hesitate to use the word *cure*. The word also implies that the immune system has healed, returned to its normal state. But we are still unraveling exactly what happens at the microscopic level during the treatment. We don't know the exact changes, although ongoing investigations are trying to figure that out. Until we know that the immune system has permanently fired all of its allergy-provoking actors, that there's no one replacing them, and that the show is over, we won't use the word *cure*. (And even when that does happen, clinicians will still probably not speak about food allergy as cured because that would require tracking people for a lifetime, which is hard to do.)

HOW CAN I ENROLL IN AN IMMUNOTHERAPY STUDY?

We are in the midst of an incredible time for food allergy research. The days when the condition was considered a fringe problem tackled by fringe researchers are long gone. If you were to picture food allergy research as a nighttime map where each new study site adds a light, you would now see glowing strands stretched continuously across the country. That doesn't mean that everyone now lives within a convenient drive to a clinical trial. But the lights are getting closer and closer together.

Ongoing clinical trials are continuing to explore how to use omalizumab and other biologic drugs, such as dupilumab, to speed up immunotherapy. They are studying treatments for allergies to milk, peanut, meat, shellfish, tree nuts, egg, wheat, and other foods. There is the OUTMATCH study by CoFAR, investigating omalizumab and multi-allergen OIT, and the MOTIF (Monitoring T Cells in Food Allergy) study investigating immunotherapy for shrimp and cashew, also funded by the NIAID.

Finding studies investigating new treatments for food allergy is not difficult. Every clinical trial receiving funding from the

National Institutes of Health and other federal agencies is listed at clinicaltrials.gov. At the search box for "condition or disease," simply type "food allergy" and every relevant study will appear. As of this writing, more than thirty food allergy trials were enrolling patients. States with study sites included Florida, California, Pennsylvania, Washington, D.C., Maryland, Colorado, Ohio, Massachusetts, Arkansas, Idaho, North Carolina, Michigan, Arizona, Alabama, and Illinois. Immunotherapy trials are also under way in Germany, Denmark, Spain, England, Iceland, the Netherlands, Ireland, France, Austria, Israel, and Australia.

The first step in identifying a possible study is to speak with your physician or allergist. A medical professional will be able to help you navigate the process of finding a trial and contacting an investigator to see if you qualify for it. Your doctor can also review the host of crucial considerations surrounding clinical trial participation. Are you willing to commit for the full duration of the study? Is your family in support of this decision? Are you prepared for the occurrence of side effects? Are there any other risks? What is your goal?

That last question is important. On the surface, the chief reason for seeking a strictly experimental treatment is because it may be better than any other available option. But from a strictly ethical standpoint, the chief reason for enrolling in a clinical trial should be to help advance the research. Therapies under investigation are by definition unproven. That means there is absolutely no guarantee that the experimental treatment will be better than either the control arm of the study (usually the current standard treatment) or what is available through a doctor. For this reason, the ethical committees governing clinical trials insist that patients be made aware that participating in a trial is not synonymous with benefiting from a clinical trial. Participants typically sign consent forms acknowledging their awareness of the purpose of the study, an ethical requirement that helps ensure that anyone undergoing an experimental treatment knows the aim of the study.

That doesn't mean people should completely erase from their

minds the possibility that the clinical trial may improve their health. With food allergy, we know the only other option to an experimental treatment is avoidance. And we know that avoidance will never improve a person's tolerance of a food allergy; all it will do is help them circumvent an allergic reaction. This equation will change as the FDA approves food allergy medications in coming years. When all allergists have access to proven, standardized regimens and the confidence to offer them to their patients, then the choice between an approved treatment and an experimental one will entail different considerations. But for now, although some allergists do offer immunotherapy in private practice (and we recommend caution before taking this route—more on that below), the vast majority of treatments are done in the setting of a clinical trial.

Inquiring about joining a clinical trial is as straightforward as it sounds. Many studies have wait lists, so it's good to be mentally prepared for that possibility. And every study has its own eligibility criteria, requirements that participants must meet in order to be considered. These criteria may pertain to age, prior treatments, allergy type, or other health issues, to name a few. A careful review of the protocol will help you and your physician determine if a study is a match for you, but often it's worth contacting the investigator team to be sure. Even if you aren't a match for the study you are calling about, it may help to be on the radar of the research team, because new studies are always in the works.

When it comes to finding and joining a study, the message essentially boils down to the well-worn phrase: it never hurts to ask. Identifying trials is simple, contacting researchers is simple, and finding out if you are eligible to participate is simple. Truly, there is nothing to lose—except possibly your food allergy.

Questions to Ask if You're Considering Immunotherapy for Yourself or Your Child

Questions for parents of children with food allergy and adults with food allergy to ask themselves:

- Can I commit to a years-long process? How will it affect my family?

- Am I (or my child) prepared to handle allergic reactions as doses are increased?

- Do I want to be freed from the threat of anaphylaxis? Do I want this for my child?

- Do I want to be able to eat my current allergen(s) without fearing an allergic reaction? Do I want this for my child?

- How much will treatment cost? Will insurance pay? Why or why not?

- How far do I need to travel for periodic increases in doses?

- Is my child ready to go through this process?

- If the therapy is effective, am I (or my child) prepared to maintain my allergy-free status by regularly eating small amounts of the former allergen?

Questions to ask the doctor:

- Are you board-certified in allergy and immunology?

- Do you have a trained team that understands food allergy immunotherapy?

- Is the product you will treat me with safe? Does it have contaminants like *E. coli* or salmonella? Does it contain the right proteins for my food allergy? Are the proteins degraded? Will the dose remain stable in the refrigerator or if it's cooked?

- Will you tell me the exact dose of proteins you are administering?

- Will you share the details of your treatment protocol with me?

- Are you using published techniques from a peer-reviewed, randomized clinical trial?

- How will you be sure that you are treating me for all the foods I am allergic to?

- Will you be available 24/7 for my calls?

- Will you share my information so that if I require a visit to the emergency room, I can inform the doctor about my immunotherapy treatment?

- Does your clinic have a psychologist that works with families?

- Does your clinic have a nutritionist?

- How do you know I (or my child) actually need this therapy?

- Will you do a food challenge after this is done to make sure that the immune system can now tolerate higher amounts of the allergen?

CAN I TRY IMMUNOTHERAPY IF I'M NOT IN A STUDY?

Unfortunately this question does not have a simple answer. At the moment, we don't have standardized immunotherapy regimens—that's what all the clinical trials are for. There are private allergists offering immunotherapy, but these specialists may be hard to find and the treatment must be paid for out of pocket. Many private allergists are experienced with controlling the quality of protein allergens—a vital part of immunotherapy—but many aren't. At some private clinics, patients are not told the exact milligrams of protein they're being given (this measurement is not the same as the milligrams of powder, which contains the protein and other substances). The clinicians may not verify that the protein they're about to provide is even going to help.

Some offer immunotherapy using flours and powders, which can be disguised in other foods, but may not confirm the absence of contaminants, such as salmonella, *E. coli,* or fungus, in the product or even the dose. Sometimes an individual may be offered immunotherapy without an oral food challenge proving that they have a food allergy in the first place. In short, rigorous evidence justifying the techniques used in a private setting may be lacking.

Many allergists are understandably hesitant about offering a treatment that they know will provoke allergic reactions. As the new era for food allergy care emerges, more allergists will be ready to add immunotherapy to their repertoire. But medicine as a practice is cautious by nature. Healthcare professionals want evidence. They want to see the data and an FDA-approved product first. Research results that support immunotherapy are emerging regularly and soon will reach the critical mass needed for a treatment to enter routine clinical care. Until that happens, immunotherapy may not be done by most allergists.

Private IT clinics are now appearing. These clinics are different from seeing a specialist who cares for all types of allergies; rather, they are stand-alone offices offering only immunotherapy. Having seen the gap between the powerful outcomes from clinical trials and the continued reluctance to embrace treatment as an option for food allergy, some entrepreneurs have taken matters into their own hands.

We predict that as IT gains popularity and widespread acceptance, private clinics will become increasingly common. As we see it, the stark data and impressive results from clinical trials should lead to regulatory approvals that make IT widely accessible. Still, more research is needed to ensure patient safety. Any clinic performing food allergy therapy should use published procedures based on work by established research centers. The protein dosing needs to be very scientific and trained staff must be available 24/7. A healthy dose of skepticism could save you from a potentially unhealthy dose of allergen.

CHOOSING AVOIDANCE

Developing a food allergy is not a choice; treatment is. Sticking with avoidance is absolutely fine, and no one should feel pressured to pursue any kind of intervention. Some people aren't able to commit to the arduous, months-long process of immunotherapy. For others, the idea of deliberately consuming a food that you have feared for all your life is a difficult prospect to swallow. Parents instruct their food-allergic children to stay away from peanuts or eggs or dairy at all costs. Packaged foods are hazardous; danger lurks at every birthday party and bake sale. And now that child is supposed to just forget about that warning and eat the very thing they've been warned to stay away from? It's not always easy.

No one—adult or child—should feel pressured to try immunotherapy. Children who are old enough to know what's happening may not be ready. As we'll come to in a later chapter, food allergy is tied to strong psychological patterns that are not simple to undo. Like a magician pulling a scarf from a hat, tugging on one end of a food allergy may unravel a host of unexpected issues that no one knew were attached to the condition. Sometimes a person needs time to become ready. Other children may need a session with a mental health professional to help them overcome any emotional hurdles blocking their way to immunotherapy. Importantly, there's no expiration date on the treatment. A person who doesn't want to pursue it at 15 years old may decide differently ten years later. The treatment will work just as well then as it would have earlier. How a person decides to address their food allergy is personal and no one should feel pressured to try immunotherapy until they are ready.

A NEW WORLD

For those who do choose immunotherapy, it's good to remember that this treatment is part of a new era for food allergy. Every individual who undergoes a regimen to desensitize their immune system to a food protein is helping to move the field forward. Every up-dosing session does a bit more to convert the vision for this new era into a reality.

But being a pioneer has its ups and downs. Although thousands of people have successfully completed treatments, we don't have a decades-long history to draw from with regard to personal experiences. Friends and family may think the treatment is risky and therefore have a hard time supporting your decision. You may find yourself repeatedly in the position of telling people about a treatment they've never heard of before. Your general practitioner and allergist may not recommend joining an immunotherapy clinical trial because their job is to provide sound and proven medical advice and they may fear straying from the norm.

We are in a strange moment in history where food allergy is concerned. On the one hand, we face a perplexing rise in rates, forcing us to confront our relationship with our environment and all that still remains mysterious about our immune system. But the spike in food allergy is directly responsible for sparking this new paradigm. It has catapulted us toward a cure. We now understand so much more about what makes us vulnerable to faulty immune reactions and how to prevent that pathway. Advances in related fields—the microbiome, for example, and even cancer immunotherapy—have dramatically expanded our understanding. Those ready to walk through to the other side carry the necessary companion to all this research: the invaluable experience of the people who are living with this condition every day and who are the intended beneficiaries of the fruits of all this labor. So many clinical and laboratory researchers have dedicated their careers to finding a better way to treat food allergy. Seeing these efforts now making a difference in people's lives is the greatest gift we could ask for.

A FINAL NOTE OF CAUTION

We cannot emphasize this point enough: **Food allergy treatment should be conducted only under the careful supervision of a** healthcare professional. **Do not try immunotherapy or any other intervention at home.** Allergic reactions can switch from mild to severe in a matter of seconds. Serious reactions require serious attention. The risk of trying immunotherapy on one's own is far too great. Don't do it.

THE BOTTOM LINE

- Immunotherapy can desensitize individuals to an allergen. In most cases, a small amount of the allergen must be consumed daily to keep the allergy at bay.

- Immunotherapy entails multiple, hours-long visits to a clinic over a period of months to years.

- Allergic reactions during treatment are a common side effect of OIT.

- Improving safety is a major priority for ongoing and future clinical trials.

- Search clinicaltrials.gov to find studies you may be able to join.

Chapter 9

THE (NOT-TOO-DISTANT) FUTURE
OF FOOD ALLERGY CARE

The new drugs, devices, and technologies
transforming the future of food allergy

The underlying theme of this book is that we are entering a new time for food allergy. Researchers around the world have contributed to a mounting pile of evidence behind a breakthrough program called immunotherapy to reverse the condition (covered in chapters 7 and 8). And we know more than ever about how to prevent it (covered in chapter 6). Thousands of people have already watched their allergy to various food proteins disappear. Many of these individuals can now freely eat foods that were once forbidden. Many more have reached the point where an accidental exposure no longer poses a threat. For an allergy researcher, few moments are more gratifying than watching children taste their first nut-filled snack or their first slice of pizza.

But the dawn of this powerful program has also lit up a vast landscape of undiscovered territory. A growing number of academic researchers are focusing their laboratories and clinics on illuminating the hidden secrets of the immune system and using them to the advantage of food allergy patients everywhere. And more and more companies are realizing that the large population of people diagnosed with food allergy makes for both a worthy cause and a tantalizing market. What all of this means for people living with food allergy is that the range of treatment regimens, medications, devices, and other technology is transforming as we speak. Within five to ten years, this world will likely look very different from today. Alfred Schofield, the physician who successfully treated his egg-allergic patient with egg back in 1908, would be stunned by the technological advances of the past few decades. But fairly soon, the field of food allergy might be unrecognizable to even current pioneers.

This chapter travels through this new territory. We'll look at the innovative devices now in the works and the drugs making their way through the research and development pipeline. We'll also dive into the latest laboratory investigations of the how and why of food allergy, crucial inquiries that could lead to ever more meaningful advances. Some of this tour involves technical science. Some of it seems more like science fiction. All of it is real and potentially important. As with any future-looking forays, there are no guarantees. We aren't wearing our rose-tinted glasses, nor should you. Progress takes time and history has proven again and again that the road from scientific question to beneficial answer is rarely short and straight. Still, we are excited and enthusiastic about the variety of ongoing projects, the dedication of those behind it, and the significance this work could have not only for people already diagnosed with food allergy but also for those who may now live without ever being affected by it.

CRACKING THE NUT

Many researchers have made an extraordinary effort to stop peanut allergy. But what if we could stop the peanut from causing allergy in the first place? That's the thinking behind the effort to create a hypoallergenic peanut. Strip the legume of its problematic parts, the thinking goes, and voilà! No more peanut allergy.

It's a tempting idea, and not a new one. Intrepid researchers have tried pulsing peanuts with ultraviolet light, firing gamma rays at them, and boiling them for half a day in the hope of making this beloved food less allergenic. A significant breakthrough arrived when researchers identified several peanut proteins that trigger an allergic reaction. These proteins—Ara h1, Ara h2, Ara h3, and Ara h6—all trigger immune system processes that end with allergic symptoms. One attempt, reported several years ago, used enzymes to break down some of these proteins in the peanut. Researchers then at North Carolina Agricultural and Technical State University created an enzyme solution that they used to remove the shell and skin from roasted peanuts, thereby reducing the amount of Ara h1 to undetectable levels and the amount of Ara h2 by 98 percent. Skin prick tests conducted with the altered legumes showed them to be far less allergenic than their ordinary counterparts (the technology was commercially licensed in 2014, but no further information is available). A team in Alabama has tried eliminating the gene encoding Ara h2, which appears to be the strongest allergen, from the peanut genome. The group created a genetically altered peanut plant and showed that IgE antibodies targeting peanut had a harder time binding to the object of their disaffection.

A more recent attempt focuses on CRISPR/Cas9, the genome editing technology that has crept into mainstream news over the past few years. The technology enables scientists to alter genes both inexpensively and easily, a capability that has brought all manner of fantastic possibilities within reach, from eradicating cancer to making disease-resistant crops. In the world of food allergy, CRISPR/Cas9 could be used to permanently change the genes encoding allergenic proteins. With their identity thus altered, the immune system would no longer attack them.

That's the thinking, at least. Peggy Ozias-Akins, a molecular geneticist at the University of Georgia, isn't sure a hypoallergenic peanut is feasible. "I would never say 'allergy-free,'" she told *Scientific American* in 2016. Removing all the genes responsible for all the allergenic proteins—at least seventeen have been identified by now—in the peanut genome is a huge undertaking and probably impossible. And geneticists don't know everything these genes encode. Stripping out the problematic proteins could also make the plant less nutritious, less tasty, or unable to fight disease.

The idea of a hypoallergenic peanut is risky. We haven't set a clear limit on how much of a reaction is acceptable, and because allergic reactions to peanut can easily veer toward serious, we wouldn't want to push a peanut as being allergy-free unless we were sure; the consequences of being wrong are too great. And as Ozias-Akins has pointed out, keeping the hypoallergenic crop separate from a regular crop is no easy feat. The plants are pollinated by insects, which fly. There's no way to stop a pollinator from traveling between a wild peanut plant and a lab-made plant without allergenic proteins. And the room for error between the fields and the supermarket could push even the most relaxed allergy parent into a panic.

All this skepticism doesn't mean an altered peanut is out of reach. The peanut genome was fully sequenced in 2019, a huge step toward isolating genes relevant to allergy. But creating a plant that is *less* allergenic may be a more realistic goal than creating one that is completely hypoallergenic. Hortense Dodo at the University of Alabama has patented her process for eliminating the three most infamous allergenic proteins (Ara h1, Ara h2, and Ara h3). In 2018, she described her genetically engineered peanut plant as "hypoallergenic straight from the fields." She envisions that the food industry could use her modified peanut, so that accidental encounters are less likely to be fatal. Scientists with the U.S. Department of Agriculture and North Carolina State University have eliminated allergenic protein from peanut plants through breeding. A genetically modified peanut plant that triggered only a mild allergic reaction could be a welcome addition for many allergy sufferers. And with the unprecedented science of CRISPR/Cas9, it is truly impossible to know what may come to pass.

NEW GENES

Another possibility emerging from the realm of genetics focuses on the other side of the food allergy equation: the human immune system. Researchers at the University of Queensland in Australia have been trying to undo the immune programming with gene therapy. They want to make the immune system forget that it ever recognized a food protein as an enemy. This notion is grounded in science. Immune cells do have a memory of sorts, though it's more akin to muscle memory than to waxing nostalgic. Like fingers dancing across a keyboard to find the notes without our conscious guidance, immune system cells remember their reactions to different substances. And similar to people themselves, these cells are stubborn about changing their opinions.

The Australian researchers believe that it's possible to mess with this wiring by introducing a new gene. The approach focuses on stem cells in the blood. After extracting them from the body, researchers add a gene that regulates how the body reacts to an allergen. The altered stem cells are then put back into the body. The new blood cells produced by these treated cells then switch off the allergic response present in specific immune system cells. The researchers, led by immunologist Ray Steptoe, succeeded in shutting down allergic reactions in animals. He hopes to improve the method to the point that a single injection could erase the memory of an allergen from the immune system entirely. To his mind, people living with lethal food allergens would be the ideal population for the treatment. But before that can come to pass, studies will have to show that the approach works as well in people as it does in animals.

SEARCHING FOR A CAUSE

We have traveled an incredible distance in the past few decades. We understand the fundamental mechanics of the immune system response to allergens. We have accrued vital knowledge about environmental factors that likely make us more vulnerable to food allergy. We have ways to prevent food allergy, and programs to reverse it.

But we still have a long way to go in unraveling the precise sequence of events that lead the immune system to react against a food protein in the first place. And we still don't fully understand the reason for the reaction. Why does the human body develop allergy? Why has this trait evolved? Is there a purpose to the response? Answering these questions isn't just an exercise in curiosity. It could help us cure the disease.

CRISPR technology could be instrumental in this pursuit. A group of researchers who are part of the Food Allergy Science Initiative at the Broad Institute are using this tool to find out which of our genes do what job when the body cultivates an immune response. CoFAR and the Immune Tolerance Network, both at the National Institutes of Health, are a group of centers across the United States working together to try to answer many questions about the biology of food allergy, such as:

- How does the immune system sense the presence of an allergen?

- What immune cells are involved in the response that we haven't yet identified?

- What don't we understand yet about why food allergy occurs? What is the body's goal with an allergic reaction?

- What gut cells are part of food allergy development and subsequent reactions?

- How exactly does the gut microbiome factor into food allergy?

HANDHELD

The laboratory science advancing our understanding of food allergy is crucial. Making strides in prevention and treatment—even broaching the idea of a cure—depends on the incremental contributions to science from painstakingly careful experiments conducted all over the world. There's no way around the fact that science takes time. Progress can happen in a leap, but that leap may depend on a decades-long running start.

Many people have their minds on finding faster ways to improve the lives of people living with food allergy. This is the realm of gadgets. Sensors, bracelets, scanners, and innovative drug delivery methods are all in the works. The plethora of emerging products shows just how far food allergy has come in gaining the attention of entrepreneurs. To be sure, not everything in the product pipeline is reliable or even viable. But a few of these new offerings are gems that could absolutely make life safer and easier for food allergy sufferers and their families.

Epinephrine Advances

Many families struggle with epinephrine. Carrying two injectors can be cumbersome and expensive. Older children feel self-conscious about the bulky item and may be less likely to carry it in a pocket because of that. And then there's the injection itself. The idea of sticking a needle into someone else's body isn't one that everyone is comfortable with from the get-go. Caregivers often need training. Children have to learn to inject themselves in case of emergency. One company is creating a nasal spray form of epinephrine that could sidestep some of these issues. First and foremost, the nasal spray avoids the need to inject the drug when an allergic reaction sets in. The spray, currently named BRYN-NDS1C, is designed to be portable and easy to use. In early 2019, after pilot studies showed a low dose of the new formulation to work just as well as injectable epinephrine, the FDA granted the product "fast track designation," which means that the agency recognizes that it serves an unmet medical need and agrees to review any study data quickly so that patients can benefit as soon as possible. The first study in people has now been completed and the results should be published in 2020.

Anaphylaxis is alarming not only because of its seriousness but because of its speed. An allergic reaction may move from mild to severe in a matter of minutes. A young child who is alone when symptoms begin may not be strong enough to use an epinephrine needle effectively. Or it may take too long for a child who realizes he or she needs help to actually find assistance. Given the profusion of wearables, it was only a matter of time before someone found a way to use the technology for food allergy.

Aibi is a bracelet that senses changes in histamine levels and signals adult caregivers when a child is in the early stages of anaphylaxis. The wearable alerts whatever other device it's linked up to—a parent's phone, a school nurse's phone—of an allergy emergency, showing a map between the child, the nearest shot of epinephrine, and the location of the recipient. If the device becomes a reality, it could help relieve some of the burden and worry that food-allergic children tend to shoulder, and give parents some extra peace of mind. Project Abbie, a product in development by the Wyss Institute of Harvard University, is similar in both name and purpose. Engineers, software developers, and physicians at Boston Children's Hospital are creating a wearable that monitors the bodily changes associated with allergic reactions. If the device detects symptoms of anaphylaxis (such as the release of histamine), it alerts the wearer and sends a message to a caregiver's phone. An accompanying device would deliver epinephrine automatically, without requiring the jab of a needle. The product, currently in development, is named after Abbie Benford, who died from anaphylaxis in 2013, a few days before her sixteenth birthday. Her parents began a fund for the project to honor her memory, hoping to help other families avoid the same fate.

Ingredient Sensors

Imagine having a device that can scan your dinner plate and alert you to the presence of your allergens. It's an idea that a few start-up companies have had, and the race is on to bring a handy, accurate, and affordable product to market.

An invention called Nima is the furthest along in terms of

availability. This triangular-shaped gadget is about the size of a wallet and currently comes in two varieties: peanut and gluten (each costs $229). A sample of food inserted into a small cylinder is ground up and then mixed with chemicals that isolate the protein from the rest of the food. Antibodies infused into a test strip sitting inside the capsule adhere to the protein, if it's present in the sample. An electronic sensor signals if the antibodies in the test strip react with any proteins. Although the gluten sensor was created mainly for people with celiac disease, an autoimmune condition, people with allergies to wheat, barley, or rye could also make use of it because these foods all contain gluten.

According to U.S. regulation, a food must contain less than 20 parts per million (ppm) of gluten in order to be considered gluten free, so the sensor is designed to detect 20 ppm or higher. In a study published in March 2019, researchers tested the ability of Nima to correctly detect the presence of gluten in samples of salad dressing, yogurt, vinegar, chocolate, butter, cheese, burger patty, ice cream, soup, prepared dough, pasta, granola, several types of flour, several types of nuts, flaxseeds, buckwheat, a mix of spices and some other items, gluten-free bread, gluten-free bread spiked with gluten, and several other items, for 447 tests in total. The device was 99 percent accurate at detecting gluten at a concentration of 20 ppm or higher. It failed to sense the protein in 3 tests, erroneously reported gluten in 10 tests where there was none, and delivered an error message in 31 of the tests. In a 2018 study, the device had a harder time detecting gluten at 20 ppm in one type of pasta but worked for 63 of 72 other food samples. The accuracy improved at 30 ppm and still more at 40 ppm.

These findings are impressive, but may also be misleading. As journalist Alex Shultz explained in a thorough review of Nima in *The Verge* in 2019, if the sensor detected gluten at levels below the standard threshold of 20 ppm, then that test was counted as a favorable result. But if the sensor failed to detect gluten below that concentration, then that failure was acceptable, since the concentration was below the standard threshold. A consumer reviewing the data would have no way of knowing nitty-gritty details like this without a very careful reading of the published paper, which very few consumers are likely to do. Researchers traced back some of the inaccuracy reported in the published data to one particular type of pasta that the sensor had a hard time with. But as *The Verge* report correctly pointed out, people who must avoid gluten would need to be assured the sensor works on all foods.

Unlike for the gluten sensor, no peer-reviewed data are available for the peanut sensor. Without a peer-reviewed study, we have no way of knowing how accurate it is. Often a device like this gets validated by an independent, uninvolved third party—someone with no stake in its success or failure. That approach ensures that bias in favor of the product doesn't influence the outcome. Two outside tests of the peanut sensor were conducted—reporting a 99.2 percent and a 98.7 percent accuracy rate—but one study was done by a lab with unclear credentials and the other used food samples prepared by Nima, introducing the possibility for bias. With Nima, the extent of outside testing is unclear.

The error rate is also troubling. It's impressive that a device can actually tell us whether a food contains a particular protein. But if it fails to detect that protein in one out of every five samples, then people with food allergy can't really rely on it. Conversely, if the sensor mistakes proteins in foods that contain no peanut or gluten whatsoever, then it also falls short of its promise.

Regulatory authorities don't necessarily help here. It's important to know that the FDA doesn't have an approval process for devices like this, as it does for new drugs, so they are free from regulatory oversight. Private companies can begin selling their wares before a rigorous study is published or even without such a study ever being conducted.

That means we may be buying a device—and more important, relying on it—without peer-reviewed data supporting its use. Peer review means that scientists with expertise in the relevant area read the study and deemed it sound (or asked for clarification and more information) before it was published. Scientific journals rely on peer review to verify that a study was conducted well, that any statistical analyses hold up, and that the conclusions make sense. Skipping this step between the laboratory and the shopping cart means we don't really know if a product is trustworthy.

Also, medical authorities haven't agreed on an acceptable concentration of peanut for a food to contain before it's considered hazardous to people allergic to it. There is no established standard for peanut equivalent to the 20 ppm considered safe for gluten. Whether there should even be a minor allowance as there is for gluten is an unsettled and controversial matter in the world of food allergy. And a failure to detect gluten or peanut in any sample from a serving of food doesn't guarantee that the entire dish is free of the allergen.

This doesn't mean Nima has no place in food allergy care. There are peer-reviewed data on the gluten-free sensor and the peanut sensor. The company has done its own testing, which is much better than no testing. Currently this device may best be used as an accompaniment to other precautionary measures. Restaurant customers with food allergies should always make sure that the server is fully aware of any foods that must not touch theirs. In food allergies, as in life, there is no substitute for taking responsibility for one's own needs.

Other Food Sensors

More allergen-sensing devices are on the way. Researchers at Harvard University have created a keychain device called iEAT, a convenient acronym for integrated exogenous antigen testing. The group reported the initial success of their invention in the journal *ACS Nano* in 2017. The portable system contains an allergen extraction kit, an analyzer that uses magnets and electrodes to detect the presence of an allergen, and a smartphone app that shows the results. The group tested five allergens—milk, egg, peanut, hazelnut, and wheat—at incredibly small concentrations, including less than 0.1 mg/kg of gluten, lower than the threshold set by regulators. The report also listed the cost of each component to support their claim that the device would cost just $40. iEAT is now in development by a private company that hopes to bring it to market within five years. A few years ago, a college student in the UK created a portable tester for lactose using a color-changing strip imbued with lactase enzyme, which reacts with the milk protein. The approach is similar to a pregnancy test. Imogen Adams, the student who designed the device, which she called Ally, planned to work on test strips for other allergens as well as one for meat that vegetarians could use. The device is not yet commercially available.

Yet another approach uses a technology called molecularly imprinted polymers to detect allergens. A polymer is simply a substance made of chains of the same molecule over and over. Polymers abound in both nature and lab-made materials. Wool, nylon, and the cellulose used to make paper are a few examples, but the list is long and vast and includes many proteins. With this technology, templates in the shape of specific protein molecules—namely, allergens—are used to create cavities on a very thin piece of film, which is attached to a circuit board. If an allergen is present in a sample of food, the protein molecule will match up with the allergen-shaped cavity. The circuit board senses the change, which sends an electronic signal. That signal turns up as an immediate alert on the keychain device. According to the company, an in-house test of the device, called Allergy Amulet, delivered an accurate reading on the presence or absence of an allergen at a concentration of 10 parts per million within 90 seconds when it was tested on fifty cupcakes. The company plans to have the device tested by a third party before making it available for purchase (it will cost between $150 and $250) in late 2020.

Other technology takes advantage of the electromagnetic spectrum, the wavelengths of energy emitted by radio waves, visible light, microwaves, and everything else we see, hear, and touch. A mouselike scanner called TellSpec fires a beam of light at a food, which excites the molecules inside, causing them to vibrate, much the same way our skin becomes warm when the sun shines on it. These vibrating molecules emit back their own photons. The scanner counts the number of photons per wavelength coming from each vibrating molecule and separates these into a spectrum, from least to most photons per wavelength. It's like a rainbow, made not of color but of the energy from different food molecules. This readout is sent to a smartphone, which sends it to the cloud—that great data storehouse in the sky—where each stripe of the rainbow is identified. Every food has a unique energy signature, making it possible to determine ingredients according to the photons they emit, the same way it's possible to identify people by their fingerprints. Within a few seconds, the cloud sends back a list of nutrients, allergens, and whatever else the food contains. The smartphone screen becomes a package label, noting the presence of gluten, egg, and other important information (it also lists the amount of carbohydrates, proteins, and fats and other data pertinent to health). And the data from the scan is saved in the cloud for future use, enabling the system to become more effective for all users over time. Fire the beam at a slice of cake and a few seconds later you'll know whether it's as nut-free as the package claims.

One of the lead developers behind TellSpec, Isabel Hoffmann, envisions creating a global "map" of what people are eating across the world and linking that with health information. That could prove useful for understanding the role of a diverse diet in the prevention of food allergy. The accuracy of the device could also hold packaged food manufacturers to account, as the scanner would reveal any ingredients not stated on the label. Such information comes at a price, though. The scanner costs about $1,900. Using the cloud to collect and store data costs a few hundred dollars per year. These prices may mean this particular device is more applicable to businesses needing to ensure that they are providing accurate information to their customers. (The scanner can also test for freshness, ripeness, and sweetness, among other qualities, which means it might be useful for supermarkets.) Still, for food allergy families with the means to purchase the device, it could prove a useful aid for preventing accidental exposure. A similar device, SCiO, is a mini sensor that also uses light to uncover the chemical makeup of a food, but this product is more geared toward researchers out in the field than a peanut-allergic child at a restaurant.

PHARMACEUTICALS

The number of drugs in development is too large to cover in this book, and not all of them will make it through the most crucial stages of clinical trials. Here are a few of the works in progress that represent the direction in which food allergy care is headed.

Vaccines

The word *vaccine* conjures various impressions. Most people associate the term with the inoculations conferring long-term protection against serious illnesses given to children throughout their elementary school years. Then there's the flu vaccine, which also protects against illness but must be given annually because the pathogen shape-shifts from year to year.

In the world of food allergy, *vaccine* carries a slightly different meaning, closer to the vaccines used to treat cancer than to the ones used to thwart polio. These drugs target an immune system already geared to attack food proteins, rather than stopping it from becoming antagonistic in the first place. ARA-LAMP-Vax is one such agent. This drug treats peanut allergy using a technology known as LAMP-Vax, which works by injecting DNA encoding a food protein into the patient. Cells in the body absorb that new DNA, which is then translated into its corresponding protein—the exact protein that triggers an allergic reaction. This launches a cascade of events in the immune system that disrupts its prior response. Instead of IgE antibodies hurling themselves at the food protein, the immune system sends cells that treat the substance as a friend. That rewriting could be accomplished in as few as four shots of vaccine and without exposing the patient directly to the allergen, thus avoiding the risk of anaphylaxis as a side effect of treatment.

Results from studies in mice gave researchers reason to think ARA-LAMP-Vax could be effective in treating peanut allergy, and the drug is now moving through clinical trials. A phase 1 study, funded by grant money and the drugmaker, is testing the safety of the drug by treating adults who are allergic to peanuts with either four doses of the compound or four doses of a placebo. A study to test the effectiveness of the vaccine will follow if the results of the phase 1 trial show the drug to be safe and potentially beneficial.

Another vaccine, PVX108, developed by Robyn O'Hehir and her colleagues in Australia, uses fragments of the allergen protein specifically engineered to avoid mast cells and basophils—the immune cells that launch allergic reactions—to desensitize the immune system. The vaccine has passed safety testing, and the next phase of clinical trials is now under way.

Gene Therapy

The addition of omalizumab to immunotherapy appears to speed up the desensitization process. Omalizumab is a monoclonal antibody that blocks the allergy-triggering IgE antibodies from attaching to the food protein they're targeted against. But the drug does have limitations. Namely, it can be used for just a few weeks, it's expensive, and it must be given by injection. Researchers at Weill Cornell Medicine wondered if they could improve the process with gene therapy. They took a segment of the genetic sequence from the monoclonal antibody used in omalizumab and inserted it into a virus. When they injected that virus into peanut-allergic mice, the animals became rapidly desensitized to peanuts. As genetic medicine specialist Ronald Crystal put it, the technique uses the virus as a "Trojan horse." Animal studies are only very rough barometers for how an approach might work in humans, so it's too soon to say if our own immune systems would fall for that particular Trojan horse. But the research is certainly worth watching.

A Plethora of Other Approaches

The quest to prevent and treat food allergy, coupled with stunning advances in our understanding of the human immune system, has spurred so many creative approaches to treatment. A primary challenge with immunotherapy is the fact that by its very definition, it prompts allergic reactions. Some groups are trying immunotherapy using modified versions of the allergens in milk, peanut, and other foods to see if they decrease the amount of IgE compared to the normal allergen. Other groups are exploring the same treatment but with peptides, which are smaller than proteins and less likely to provoke IgE antibodies into action.

Another attempt to lessen the allergic reactions that occur as a side effect of immunotherapy is by using nanoparticles containing peanut extract instead of pure peanut powder. In a preliminary study, mice treated with these nanoparticles (which are simply minuscule molecules) exhibited milder allergic reactions to peanuts compared to mice treated with the standard approach.

Dendritic cells, part of the immune system, can introduce antigens—the foreign structures that antibodies are trained to recognize as friend or foe—to other immune cells as a form of protection. These cells "talk" to T cells, delivering the message that a protein is safe. And because dendritic cells can field multiple allergens at once, new approaches involving them are particularly appealing for the treatment of people allergic to more than one food. Small amounts of the relevant food proteins may be all that is needed to resolve the allergies.

A new antibody called etokimab targets an immune molecule called interleukin-33 (IL-33), which launches a cascade of events when an allergen enters the body. In a recent study at Stanford, we randomized 20 adults with severe peanut allergy to either an antibody that inhibits IL-33 or a placebo. Two weeks later, 11 of the 15 people in the treatment group could eat 275 milligrams of peanut protein (about one peanut), whereas none of the placebo group could do so. It's still early days in the investigation of this drug and others like it.

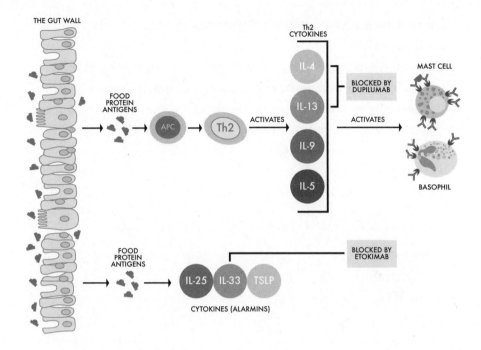

New drugs in development for the treatment of food allergy tackle the immune system in different ways. The antibody dupilumab stops interleukin (IL)-4, -13, -9, and -5 from activating the mast cells and basophils that IgE is attached to, which in turn stops IgE from triggering the release of histamines and other symptom-triggering chemicals. Another antibody, etokimab, stops the activation of IL-33, another trigger for IgE activation.

Other biologic drugs are also under investigation. Dupilumab is similar to omalizumab and is being combined with immunotherapy in the same way. The drug is now in phase 2 and 3 clinical trials. A long list of experimental drugs, all in the same category, is following close behind, including mepolizumab, reslizumab, benralizumab, lebrikizumab, and tralokinumab. Each of these biologic agents works by targeting some aspect of the immune response pathway between the protein entering the body and anaphylaxis. It's possible that at some point, a monthly shot of antibody will be all we need to keep the immune system from reacting to an allergen. Researchers are also working on a way to disguise allergenic proteins as they enter the body. Hidden in this way, the protein could escape the initial allergic response and instead infiltrate the immune system and induce tolerance.

The proliferation of biologic drugs means that in five to ten years, the number of weapons we have to fight food allergy in the clinic will likely dwarf what we have today. But for now, actual exposure to the antigen itself appears to be the only way to resolve food allergy more permanently in some individuals.

SOME NEW THERAPIES ON THE HORIZON		
DRUG TYPE	TRIED IN FOOD ALLERGY	CLINICAL TRIAL PHASE
BIOLOGICAL INHIBITOR		
Anti IL-4R	Yes	2
Anti IL-4	Not yet	
Anti IL-13	Not yet	
Anti IL-33	Yes	2
VACCINE		
LAMP-Vax	Yes	2
Peanut epitope	Yes	1
Aluminum peanut	Yes	2
OTHER		
Multi-allergy OIT	Yes	2
Microbiome	Yes	1
Nanoparticle	Not yet	

ALLERGY-PREVENTING TREATS

The revelation that early introduction of common allergens is better than waiting until a child is several years old has led some entrepreneurs to seize that most inevitable of opportunities: snacks. It's one thing to recommend that babies try fish by the time they're 1 year old; it's another thing for a busy parent to make sure that happens, especially if the child is a fussier eater. Preventing multiple food allergies is better than preventing just one, so a mixture of proteins is helpful. And there is always—always—a need for a handy, crunchy finger food.

Enter the "allergy protection system." Packaged foods made from small amounts of common allergens may be a reliable and simple way to make sure a child is exposed to almost all foods early on. A product called Spoonful One comes in a powder form that can be mixed into baby food, and also comes in puffs that can be picked up by little fingers practicing their dexterity (disclosure: Kari is a co-founder of Before Brands, the company that makes Spoonful One). The foods contain proteins from peanut, soy, almond, cashew, hazelnut, pecan, pistachio, walnut, wheat, oat, milk, egg, cod, shrimp, sesame, and salmon, all contained in the equivalent of about a teaspoon of powder. In tests conducted by researchers at Northwestern University's Feinberg School of Medicine, 705 infants between 5 and 11 months old were randomized to receive either the "food mix" from Before Brands or a placebo. None of the infants who completed the mix arm of the study had any allergic reactions, suggesting that the product was a safe way to expose babies to these crucial proteins. Moreover, those that underwent a food challenge had no reactions. Giving many food proteins together had a better effect on the immune system. Other companies are also offering foods for prevention. A supply that provides enough exposure during the first few months of life costs about $2 per day.

Any infant can start products like these, whether or not they have a family history of food allergy and whether or not they have eczema. Regardless of the product, be sure that the proteins have been tested for stability and are free from contaminants like bacteria and fungi. Infants should not eat these foods if they already have an allergy diagnosis from a board-certified allergy specialist. Evidence from early introduction studies suggests that eating products with many food proteins daily for about a year achieves optimal protection against food allergy.

APPS

Smartphone apps are fertile ground for developers wishing to improve the lives of people with food allergy. A couple of them have emerged as particularly useful. Rescufy places a button on the home screen that can be tapped if an emergency arises. This tool means a person doesn't have to unlock their phone during an allergic reaction, and tapping the button sends out a message to emergency responders and personal emergency contacts containing the user's allergy and GPS location, along with medical and insurance information. Allerpal is designed to help parents or caregivers alert others about a child's allergies. The app allows the user to upload information about the child's allergy, including how to address a reaction, and emergency contact information. The user can then send an alert to anyone else who has Allerpal—a sports coach, a friend's parents, a babysitter, a teacher. Obviously the app is effective only if the other grown-ups in a child's life also use it, but if word spreads, it could be an extremely helpful tool for food-allergic children.

This chapter is by no means comprehensive. New products are always entering the pipeline, whether at a pharmaceutical company, a snack-food start-up, or a software developer. Financial analysts predict that by 2025, the allergy treatment market will represent a $40 billion market. Food allergy accounts for just a portion of this market, but it's forecast to grow the fastest, at a rate of 8.3

percent per year. A report in late 2018 anticipated that the global peanut allergy market would grow by 90 percent from 2019 to 2023. And of course peanut is far from the only food allergy that needs to be addressed.

All of us can decide for ourselves how to think about this explosion. Some may find the link between an epidemic and profits a little shocking. Others may be inspired to see doctors at academic institutions and businesses rallying to improve the tools that food allergy families have at their disposal. We see both sides. Although we encourage families to approach new products with caution, we are also thankful to see the expanding array of treatments and other help for this very serious condition. People will select the advances that are right for themselves or their children—because the future of food allergy is one filled with options.

THE BOTTOM LINE

- Researchers are trying to create foods that are less allergenic by breeding out the most allergenic proteins, or genetically manipulating foods using techniques such as CRISPR/Cas9.

- Innovations for food allergy on the horizon include:
    - Smaller, more user-friendly epinephrine devices
    - Wearables that detect the onset of allergic reactions
    - Ingredient sensors that detect allergens in foods
    - Vaccines and biologic drugs
    - Snack foods containing food proteins that infants can eat as part of early introduction

Part III

PERSONAL AND GLOBAL PERSPECTIVES

Chapter 10

THE EMOTIONAL TOLL OF FOOD ALLERGY

*Insights and tools to end the fear, anxiety,
confusion, and frustration*

Nurse practitioner Jamie Saxena had a suspicion. She was pretty sure that the 11-year-old boy sitting in the exam room was not allergic to peanuts, even though he'd avoided them his entire life. The only way to be sure was to try an oral food challenge with him, giving him tiny but increasing amounts of peanut to see if his body reacted.

Most of the doses had been so small that she had to use peanut flour, which she mixed into pudding. No allergic symptoms appeared. Eventually the dose reached the point where he was ready to try the actual food. Saxena gave him a peanut M&M. But instead of eating it just as he'd been doing, he froze. "He could not bring the food to his mouth," says Saxena, who is part of our team at Stanford. She stood next to him as he tried. Again and again he would open his mouth, bring his hand up to his mouth, and become paralyzed with fear. He cried hysterically. "He was petrified that what we were asking him to do was going to kill him," she says.

The team of clinicians surrounding him did their best to encourage and calm him. Saxena reassured him that she was highly trained to manage allergic reactions, that she trusted in the medications, and that even if he did have an allergic reaction, that did not mean he would die.

The child eventually ate the M&M and had no reaction. He wasn't allergic. A doctor had interpreted a blood test years earlier as indicating an allergy, but the child had never tried eating a peanut. He'd lived the first 11 years of his life believing he had an allergy that in fact he did not. But although the memory remains a vivid one for Saxena, it would turn out to be not all that unusual. That paralyzing grip of fear was something she would encounter repeatedly as she ushered patients through food allergy tests and treatments.

Food allergy is stressful, to state the obvious. From the first time a child's lips swell or skin becomes dotted with hives, the fear of allergic reactions hovers just under the surface of daily life. It reaches up when a birthday invitation arrives and on school field trips. It intrudes into playdates, teenage movie outings, and first kisses. It makes parents overprotective and sometimes makes children panic. Growing up with food allergy often means moving through many psychological phases, from paralyzing paranoia to rebellious recklessness.

To make matters more difficult, many food allergy families have no idea how far from alone they are. At some point during her elementary school years, Nikki Godwin's elder child, who is allergic to several foods, began having panic attacks. That stretch of time was made more difficult by the fact that Nikki (whom we first met in chapter 5) had no idea how common this kind of response is among children with food allergies. Eventually she realized just how often other children had similar experiences. "It blew my mind that I've never heard of it," she says.

No family with food allergy should feel alone in their struggle to cope. In recent years, allergists and pediatricians have become much more cognizant of this emotional toll. In fact, therapists have begun specializing in the unique issues faced by food allergy families. This shift is spurred in part by mounting evidence about how food allergy influences the decisions, outlook, and experiences of a person diagnosed with the condition and those of the people who care most about them.

It's one thing to say that food allergy curbs family life. But what, exactly, does it change? A group of pediatric allergists and psychologists from the University of Maryland asked 87 caregivers about how their child's food allergy affected meals, social activities, school, extracurricular activities, and other aspects of raising a family. Most of the participants said the food allergy affected meal preparation, including grocery shopping and grabbing snacks on the run. Nearly 80 percent said it altered what restaurants they go to—16 percent of the respondents said they don't even go out to eat because of the food allergy—and nearly 60 percent said it affected their decisions about letting their child go play at a friend's house. Although not all of these changes translated into feeling stressed, the more food allergies the child had, the more stress parents reported.

A group of researchers in the UK wanted to hear from peanut-allergic children directly. They asked 20 children with peanut allergy and 20 children with diabetes (all between the ages of 7 and 12) to complete a questionnaire about their fears and concerns. The researchers also gave each child a disposable camera to take pictures illustrating how their condition affected their weekend. The questionnaire revealed that children with peanut allergy feared accidental exposure more than children with diabetes feared a hypoglycemic attack. A few of the peanut-allergic children were quite scared of this possibility. Most of them said they always had to be careful about avoiding peanuts, but just half of the diabetes group said they had to maintain constant vigilance about their own diet. The peanut-allergic children had more anxiety about vacations, birthdays, and taking public transportation.

The photographs provided an interesting window, though a limited one, since the exercise was done over just one twenty-four-hour period. The children with peanut allergy took a lot of pictures of restaurants, whereas the children with diabetes commented about restaurants just twice and in a neutral way. They all took pictures of food: the peanut-allergic children because they were scared and the diabetes children because they were frustrated by their restrictive diets. When peanut-allergic children took photographs of physical activities, it was often to show that they felt limited in what they were allowed to do. They all photographed people, saying they felt comforted by others with the same condition who could therefore sympathize with them. But the peanut-allergy group also had some negative feelings about other people. "My grandma buys my brother and me sweets, but she forgets about my allergy and buys things I cannot have," one child noted. "It's really annoying." And they worried about going places where peanuts were present, like supermarkets. The study let the researchers see life through the eyes of a child with peanut allergy. "Simple tasks such as shopping or eating in a restaurant can be extremely frightening," they wrote, "even perceived as life-threatening."

One study found that children with peanut allergy were actually better at coping with the stress of their condition than were newly diagnosed adults. The adults in the study were more lax about carrying epinephrine with them and felt less in control as a result. It may be that the suddenness of the condition gives newly diagnosed adults less time to learn to cope, whereas children who grow up allergic to one food or another are used to dealing with it. Grown-ups, the researchers found, were much better at managing their children's allergies than their own.

Teenagers experience a unique set of challenges, different from those of younger children under the near-constant supervision of parents or other grown-ups. Eating outside of the home is at the center of so many social occasions for teens. If young adults with food allergy are self-conscious about asking restaurant servers about allergens in the dish they're ordering when they are with their friends, then they may not do so. A study from many years ago found that most teens who died from anaphylaxis weren't home when they ate something containing their allergen.

Researchers in New Zealand asked a group of young adults who were about to leave home for college about their awareness and perceptions of food allergy. Some said that the condition affected their lives less than people think. That finding suggests that young people with a food allergy are aware of its seriousness but may not always take the risk of exposure to heart. This pattern may be familiar to many parents of teens: recognizing the risk and the stress it causes, but preferring to take that risk rather than bother with the simple steps to eliminate it. It's a pattern summed up by the all-too-familiar phrase "I'll be fine, Mom, don't worry." Interestingly, it was the teens who didn't feel fully equipped to manage their allergy who reported the highest levels of anxiety. The ones who felt most competent reported the same level as teens without food allergy.

By now, enough data have been gathered to pinpoint the psychosocial effects of food allergy. Adjusting to food allergy immediately following a diagnosis produces some anxiety, but it's really the fear of an accidental exposure that's responsible for most of the daily stress. It can be tricky, a group of pediatricians wrote in 2016, to weigh the need for vigilance against the need to ensure that children do not become unreasonably scared. They noted that an oral food challenge can be beneficial because it resolves any lingering doubt about whether or not an allergy exists, something that other forms of testing really can't do. These pediatricians also identified what they saw as the specific psychological issues facing younger children as opposed to older children.

EARLY CHILDHOOD

Coping with food allergy during a child's earliest years is largely a matter of balance. Parents feel understandably anxious about playdates, playground outings, and other activities outside the house. Many parents forgo certain events altogether because they find preparing for them to be so stressful. They avoid restaurants; they don't travel. Some parents decide to reduce their work hours as a result of their child's food allergy.

But autonomy is a key element of childhood development. Children must slowly grow to feel more comfortable without their parents around and must become more capable of doing things on their own, one small step at a time. Food allergy parents may have a hard time with that. "It's really the opposite mind-set than the one you want to be in as a parent," says Melanie Thernstrom. Most parents of young children have the joy of introducing them to the world and encouraging them to explore. "Instead, the journey of a food allergy parent is you learn to be more and more controlled and paranoid, and you get the lesson again and again that there's no one you can trust to take care of your child," says Melanie. That anxiety, she notes, may also infect the child. Melanie and her husband eventually put a sign on their front door saying no eggs or nuts were allowed inside after weekend houseguests brought both. (She laughs now when she remembers how that deterred neighborhood Girl Scouts from trying to sell them cookies.) Food allergy parents may stay at birthday parties long after other parents have stopped doing so. They may linger at school or other places where parents don't typically hang around after drop-off. That parental behavior could lead to more separation anxiety in children temporarily. Mostly it means that parents need to teach their young child about how to be safe in the world, and they need to feel confident that the child has actually absorbed that information.

THE ELEMENTARY YEARS

In their review of the data, the researchers found that the dynamics change as children move through their single-digit years. By the time they're 8 or 9 years old, children are much more aware of the reality of their food allergy. They can become more fearful of death than when they were younger. Social situations can become more difficult. Bullying is a big issue for food-allergic children. Kim Yates, whose daughter, Tessa, was treated with immunotherapy for multiple food allergies, recalls an occasion where a classmate pretended to stumble with her lunch tray, shooting fear through Tessa about being splashed with milk—an occurrence that had landed her in the emergency room when she was less than 2 years old. Classmates occasionally taunted her by saying they'd just eaten peanut butter, so she'd better watch out. "Those types of jokes scared me," says Tessa. "I don't blame anyone for not understanding, but I was bullied." In 2017, a dairy-allergic British teenager died after a classmate teasingly flicked a piece of cheese at him.

In a study from allergy researchers at Mount Sinai School of Medicine, 80 of the 251 children surveyed said they'd been bullied at least once due to their food allergy. A year later, a follow-up survey by the same group found that three quarters of the children who'd been bullied a year earlier were still being bullied. A third said such interactions happened more than twice a month. Children with food allergy may be excluded by their classmates and teased or taunted like Tessa was. Many parents have heard stories of peers dangling dangerous foods in front of their children. These kinds of experiences can leave children deeply distressed.

TEENAGERS

As one study discussed above pointed out, the trials and tribulations of food allergy shift yet again when adolescence sets in. At this time in their lives, children start becoming responsible for managing their food allergy, and parents have to find ways to let that transition happen. That's made harder by the fact that parents and teenagers already struggle over independence and responsibility. The risk of an allergic reaction increases during this time because teenagers forget their epinephrine, take the risk of eating packaged foods without certainty of their contents, and go out to eat with their friends.

In another study, two thirds of 174 food-allergic teenagers said they'd had an allergic reaction within the last five years. Most said they would carry epinephrine while traveling, but less than half said they'd bring it to sports activities. Wearing tight clothing was also a deterrent to carrying the medication. The researchers also observed a reluctance to take epinephrine with them to friends' houses or to other social activities. Predictably, the children who took the greatest risks also had the most recent reactions. Most of the teens thought that life would be easier if their friends understood more about what it's like to have a food allergy. Adolescents are still anxious about accidental exposure; those who believe they could die from eating their food allergen report the highest levels of stress.

A study from McMaster University perfectly illustrates the conundrum of food-allergic teenagers: mothers, the study found, report their teens as having emotional and behavioral issues far more often than the teenagers themselves do. Researchers from Canada used data from a large Australian study that included 1,300 children to gauge how common emotional and behavioral issues were among food-allergic teens, and to see the difference between what mothers say and what teenagers say about themselves in this regard. They also wanted to see how these challenges change as teenagers move into young adulthood. According to their 2016 report, a third of 14-year-olds with food allergy said they had emotional and behavioral problems. But among their mothers, nearly half said their children struggled with these issues, including depression, anxiety, and attention deficit hyperactivity disorder. The researchers couldn't be certain whether the teens were under-reporting or the moms were over-reporting. But seven years later, 44 percent of the original food-allergic group said they had emotional and behavioral problems—nearly twice as many as the nonallergic group. The data made it clear that the emotional issues linked to food allergy, unlike other roller-coaster emotions of adolescence, are more likely to persist into adulthood. "These problems are not just a phase," as Mark Ferro, who led the study, put it at the time of the report. It also goes to show how differently others see us compared to how we see ourselves—and sometimes the others are right.

PERSONALITY AND FOOD ALLERGY

As is clear from this chapter already, people handle stress differently from one another. Young children are different from older children.

Parents are different from teenagers. Personality presents yet another layer to that onion. Our temperament greatly influences how we see the world and respond to whatever comes our way—including food allergy.

Psychologists have identified several personality traits, sometimes referred to as the Big Five: neuroticism, extroversion, openness, agreeableness, and conscientiousness. A host of studies have found links between personality type and how we cope with illness. For example, research suggests that people with neurotic personalities, who often have a lot of negative emotions, may have trouble adapting to their illness. They may also have more severe symptoms.

A group of psychologists in New Zealand wanted to see whether these links extend to the daily experience of food allergy. Are extroverts better at speaking up and therefore restaurants are less stressful for them? Do conscientious personality types take fewer risks or are they more anxious about unknown dangers? To find out, they asked 108 people (age 18 or over, with an average age of 40) with one or more common food allergies to complete at least five daily surveys within a two-week period. The survey collected information about their mood and stress levels and about any issues related to food allergy.

Although the sample size was relatively small, the survey found some intriguing connections. Participants with the open personality type also had a higher number of food allergies. That link doesn't necessarily mean anything—just because two measures match up doesn't mean they're connected (in the words of scientific research, correlation doesn't imply causation)—but the finding is interesting. There were no connections between personality type and the number of food allergy issues—meaning, people who tended to be on the neurotic side weren't complaining more than anyone else about allergic reactions. Rather, it was the people who were more open who voiced their issues more. They talked about having to go hungry because no safe foods were available, about frustrating experiences at the supermarket, and about the cost (financial and social) of food allergy. Extroverts—outgoing people—lamented the unkindness people sometimes exhibited about their allergy, but they felt less stressed out by food allergy issues. Agreeable people reported feeling stressed out by social occasions involving food. When allergic reactions happened, conscientious people were more affected emotionally. None of this is hard evidence about how a given person might respond to food allergy. But studies like this show us how important it is to make space for varying ways of coping with the strains of food allergy. There is always some form of coping going on when a food-allergic person is faced with a social event involving food, the school cafeteria, or just a trip to the supermarket. The issue is making sure that the coping is productive rather than destructive.

FOOD ALLERGY ANXIETY

The psychological burden of food allergy expresses itself in a multitude of ways. Jeanne Herzog, PhD, a Wisconsin-based psychologist who works often with food allergy families, notes that not all anxiety is bad. A little bit can keep us alert to danger or make us aware that something isn't right, whether internally or externally. When it comes to food allergy, anxiety can help a person stick to the rules for avoiding exposure. But it's good to know the signs of anxiety overload. Children may develop psychosomatic allergy symptoms, for example. They may cry or feel inexplicably tired. They may withdraw or become prickly. They may pick fights or, Herzog notes, try to get attention in ways that seem unhealthy.

Of course, behavior changes with age. Through age 6, children often mirror their parents' emotions, says Herzog, discovering their own independent feelings only starting at around age 7, which is also when the world outside their family starts to become important. As teenagers, children are often better able to express their feelings with some level of maturity, though this takes time and moves at different speeds for different children. Herzog also recommends that parents look through different lenses—emotional, social, and cognitive—to understand their children, as each of these follows its own development journey.

Marté Matthews, a consulting therapist at Stanford University, meets often with food allergy families participating in immunotherapy studies and in her private practice. She cautions that children with food allergy can sometimes develop complicated and problematic eating habits. She draws a distinction between feeding disorders and eating disorders. The latter category includes familiar issues such as anorexia and bulimia, which are often characterized by a misperception of how the body looks. Feeding disorders having nothing to do with looks. Rather, says Matthews, "there's a misperception of a food as being dangerous or disgusting." Food allergy anxieties may manifest as feeding disorders, a link Matthews has seen many times over. Restricting foods beyond what is necessary is the most common situation she sees. That behavior can also make parents understandably impatient because, says Matthews, "it feels exaggerated or out of proportion." That parent-child dynamic then becomes its own stressful situation.

Monitoring Anxiety in People with Food Allergies: What to Watch For

- Overly restrictive eating
- Refusal to participate in social activities
- Withdrawn, fearful, clingy, or sad
- Lack of interest in hobbies or friends
- Angry, acting out, being aggressive, and misbehaving
- Sleep problems: too much, not enough, awake in the middle of the night, and/or frequent nightmares

Families coping with food allergy need to stay vigilant, strong, and well-informed. The condition presents its fair share of challenges, which makes for a courageous and heroic demographic. And prevailing over the difficulties, whatever they may be, makes it that much easier for the next person.

IMMUNOTHERAPY AND ANXIETY

Ending the threat posed by a food allergy is beneficial in so many ways. "It has changed my life totally," says Andy Hartman, 18, a freshman at Northwestern University who underwent immunotherapy at Stanford when he was in eighth grade. He relishes family vacations that no longer revolve around keeping him safe, not having to ask about ingredients at restaurants, and being able to live in a dorm without fear. But the process included some unexpected hurdles.

One of the more unexpected emotional challenges lies with identity. For children who grow up with a food allergy, the condition often becomes part of who they are. And the more severe the allergies, the more central they are likely to be to the person's identity. Families pursuing immunotherapy often have to wrestle with that trait. Andy's mother, Kim, remembers talking about this issue when he started the treatment. "We talked about kids who lose their allergies and lose their identity," she says. Working with a therapist helped him resist that trap. Tessa remembers not wanting to admit to her parents that part of her reluctance to try immunotherapy was her attachment to the label. "Food allergies defined me," says Tessa, who was desensitized by the time she was 10. "If I got rid of them, I wouldn't have anything that made me unique or set me apart from anyone else."

Matthews says the identity of being a food allergy kid can be replaced by other identities—one of the soccer kids, say, or even the kid who beat food allergy. "That's not a fast process," she cautions. "It's an incremental process that one works on over a long period of time." For Tessa, overcoming the allergy helped her form a new identity. "Immunotherapy has essentially defined my life," she says. The confidence, freedom, and sense of safety she now has are qualities that she traces directly to overcoming the multiple food allergies that once kept her isolated and afraid.

Treating an allergy with immunotherapy can dredge up other anxieties, too. When children have been told to avoid a food for their entire lives, it's not that easy to suddenly try even the tiny amounts given at the start of the treatment. "When you're told there is a thing in the world that can kill you and then you're told you have to eat that thing, every day, for who knows how long," says Andy, "that is terrifying." Andy describes his daily tiny-dose consumption as one of the most difficult things he's ever had to do. "It wasn't something anyone could help me with," he said. His parents supported him however they could and his family tolerated the drama he insisted on making whenever he finally worked up his nerve to eat the apple-sauce or pudding or other food he'd put the nut powder into on a given day. ("I feel bad now that I drew so much attention to myself," he says.) But in the end, no one could help him actually eat the food. "It was an individual thing," says Andy.

At Stanford, we try to defuse anxiety by explaining the process. When Matthew meets with patients embarking on immunotherapy, she tells them that the treatment is not at all the same as acciden-tally eating peanut at a restaurant or getting splashed with milk. Those hazardous exposures involve higher quantities of a food and they don't occur at a hospital or a doctor's office with epinephrine and a crash cart nearby. She knows the idea of eating a food they've been told to stay away from—one that they may never have even tasted—can be extremely difficult for children and teens.

Sloan's daughter, Violet, struggled hugely with immunotherapy. She grew up allergic to all tree nuts and, when she was in fifth grade, enrolled in our first multi-allergy study. Her treatment began with shots of omalizumab, followed by a year or so of escalating doses of several different nuts. For Violet, the stretch of time between con-suming her dose and having an allergic reaction was the hardest part. "It was one or two hours of knowing I'd just had a nut," she said. She knew at some point she would throw up, but all she could do was wait. The anticipation, combined with the allergic reaction her body had to nuts—severe abdominal pain, itchiness, hives, swelling, her throat closing up—was, she says, "a lot for my 10-year-old self to handle." Taking her doses at home was equally difficult. She would eat her nuts at 5:00 P.M. every day. "And every day at five, I would cry," she says. "I was so scared."

Yet she persevered. "There was no way out but through," says Violet, now a senior in high school. The treatment worked. Now she doesn't need to worry anymore about a life-threatening reaction from an accidental exposure to nuts during her frequent weekend trips for sports. She knows that when she goes away to college, she won't die if she eats a nut. She has come to feel thankful for the process she once dreaded. "I had to grow up a bit," she says, "to realize how amazing it was."

Families with internal struggles may find this time especially fraught, says Matthews. A parent talking a child into immunotherapy may result in a messy situation for all involved. Like any pivotal moment in life, the start of treatment may unearth emotions that already existed within the family but were simmering beneath the surface. "The medical treatment of food allergy or a series of emergency room visits because of accidental exposures are going to bring out and turn up whatever those dynamics are," says Matthews.

HOW TO HELP SOMEONE WITH FOOD ALLERGY ANXIETIES

Improvements in our understanding of anxiety have led to accompanying improvements in how we deal with it. We know better coping mechanisms and we teach them to others, including schoolchildren. Mindfulness, breathing techniques, and other methods for calming anxieties are often taught in schools to help students monitor and manage their emotions better. As Jeanne Herzog puts it, "knowing

what it feels like in our bodies and knowing what our thinking process is when we're anxious or depressed" are the types of awareness
that teachers and mental health professionals who work with children now encourage.

But the emotional burden of food allergy calls for some specific
tools. As described above, young children may be faced with social
exclusion or the stigma of having to sit at the nut-free table. Older
children become aware of the potential for dying as a result of accidental exposure. All people with food allergy live with the feeling of
not having complete control over their safety. As Herzog explains,
bullying, feeling left out, vulnerability, and all the other issues specific to food allergy have ramifications. Often, says Herzog, the result is that children with food allergy grow up faster. "They have to
learn how to cope. Otherwise they will curl up in a ball and not be
able to function."

Herzog has worked with families to create what she calls emotional safety plans. These plans include coping mechanisms similar
to those often recommended for anxiety, such as mind-body methods
and cognitive behavioral therapy, tailored to the unique strains of
food allergy. Herzog works with families to accept the challenge of
the condition bravely, to empower children with knowledge, to seek
support, and to find balance. Her safety plan for young children and
teenagers includes several recommendations, including:

- Learn and follow your emergency care plan.
- Tell others about what your food allergy means to you.
- Be aware of your feelings so they protect you, not hinder
  you.
- Calm your thoughts.
- Calm your body with strategies.
- Learn all you can about yourself. Your allergy is only one
  thing about you.

For adults with food allergy, her advice is similar and adds:

- Create your normal lifestyle.
- Find your people.
- Seek support when necessary.

The typical recommendations for quelling anxiety may seem simplistic, but they work. And they are easy to teach children so that they can reach for these tools on their own. Herzog believes children with food allergy should learn how to calm themselves down and has several suggestions for doing so:

- Have a drink of water.
- Get some fresh air.
- Listen to music.
- Play!
- Pet the cat or dog, if you have one.
- Ask for a hug from someone you trust.

Parents can help calm their children using gentle touch. Belly breathing—a form of deep breathing that contracts the diaphragm, which is located between the thoracic cavity and the abdominal cavity—can also help. This technique, also called diaphragmatic breathing, can slow the heartbeat and lower blood pressure.

Herzog suggests some other practical ideas:

- Keep track of successes by writing them down.
- Create an incentive plan to help children try new foods when they are feeling fearful or resistant.

- Have a safety checklist that children can review before choosing a food to help them feel secure during meals outside the home.

- To help relieve anxiety, make relaxation a family activity.

Safety Checklist for Food-Allergic Patients Dining at Restaurants

- Can the server assure me that my allergens are not in the food I am ordering?

- Are there any ingredients that come from packaged foods in this dish?

- Have I had this food before?

- Have I eaten at this restaurant before?

- Are the grown-ups I am with aware of my food allergy?

- Do I have epinephrine with me, and is there someone who knows how to inject it in case of an emergency?

- Is the restaurant interested in ensuring that food allergens are accurately labeled on the menu?

Knowing your support team can also make a huge difference to children. With so many unknowns, it can help to be certain of who they can rely on to take their food allergy seriously. Some studies have found that children are more fearful of people who don't care about their allergy than they are of the actual allergens, notes Herzog. The anxiety is exacerbated because the risk of exposure seems higher when the people you're around seem to be either uncaring or unaware. The family of Andy Hartman's best friend when he was growing up decided to keep a nut-free home because he was there so much. "I surrounded myself with people who were so willing to help," he says. He wrestled with feeling that he was a burden to the people who went out of their way to keep him safe, but he also knows what a difference those efforts made to his childhood. Herzog suggests that children tell their peers not only that they have a food allergy but also how it feels to live with a food allergy. And although she says finding others with food allergy in your community can provide an enormous sense of support, she also emphasizes the importance of raising awareness outside of the food allergy community. "Advocate for yourself," she says, "so others can be aware and care."

Instilling a long-term view is also a good idea. For Matthew Friend, now 21, food allergy is still part of his life even though he's become desensitized through immunotherapy. An aspiring comedian, he incorporates his childhood experience with a wheat allergy into his routine. He remembers disliking cheese as a child and likes to joke with his audience that whenever he wanted food that wasn't safe for him, his mother would just tell him it had cheese in it. And having to ask a girl to brush her teeth before they kissed was, he says, "the perfect way to ensure amazing breath."

Seventeen-year-old Ariella Nelson, who was treated in Kari's clinic for a peanut allergy, says coping with a food allergy taught her to speak up. When she spent a summer away from home for a music program, she knew she had to be around other people as a safety precaution when she took her daily nut dose. That meant asking new friends if she could hang out in their room, a small request that took some boldness. "I would call myself a pretty assertive person," she says, "and I could see that coming from dealing with my tree nut allergy." Anyone who grows up with food allergy will be shaped by the experience in some way. The trick is to find a way for that shape to be one we choose, not one imposed upon us.

WHEN TO SEEK PROFESSIONAL HELP

As we talked about above, the challenges of food allergy can sometimes lead to extreme behavior. Children may restrict their eating, out of fear of accidental exposure, to the point that they risk malnutrition, a condition known as avoidant restrictive food intake. Tessa remembers being so afraid to put anything in her mouth during a weekend stay with relatives soon after a severe allergic reaction that she ate only white rice for the entire weekend. Life-threatening experiences can lead to post-traumatic stress disorder, a serious condition in its own right. Sometimes no amount of belly breathing and journaling can make a dent in the mountain of food allergy–induced stress.

Here is where mental health professionals come in. A therapist may begin by bonding and connecting with patients, understanding the issues they are grappling with as much as possible and validating the feeling that these issues are difficult. Learning and practicing coping tools is the other key component. Therapists teach many of the same strategies that Herzog recommends—calming the mind, challenging negative thinking, becoming more empowered—but sometimes it's different when a professional is leading the way.

Avoidant restrictive food disorder also requires care by other specialists. A dietitian and an occupational therapist should be consulted alongside the therapist, says Marté Matthews. This condition is a serious issue that warrants a team of people addressing it together.

Matthews often helps families pinpoint holes in a person's routine that may be contributing to feelings of vulnerability or fear. If children are old enough to carry their own epinephrine, are they? If not, what are the obstacles? How can those obstacles be dismantled? Do children speak up about their needs? Can they be trusted to ask questions or refuse food that isn't sure to be safe? Or are they likely to accept unsafe food because they think it's rude to say no? These are some of the questions that Matthews tackles regularly with food allergy families.

Power struggles between parents and food-allergic teenagers may also be dealt with best using professional help. And when dealing with food allergy uncovers other issues within the family, a psychologist can facilitate untangling these knots so that the fundamental needs of food allergy care remain unclouded by heightened emotions, resentment, and anger.

Therapy can also help parents mellow out. Watching children struggle can often lead the grown-ups in their lives to want to solve the problem. That doesn't always work, says Matthews. The birthday party that they weren't invited to is over. Mom and Dad can't stop the teasing in the cafeteria tomorrow or next week or next year. "I will help parents learn how to actively and reflectively listen to their children," says Matthews of her work with food allergy families. She'll counsel parents who are hurting for their excluded child to resist reacting when the feelings are raw. "Yes, advocate for your child," she says, "but maybe wait to send that email until you're not quite as angry." Matthews also helps families develop lists of coping skills that work within their own unique dynamic. Shooting baskets at the park, going for a walk, splashing cold water on your face—these are some of the simple measures to try. Guided imagery and deep breathing can also help. "Distraction and relaxation techniques are two sides of the toolbox we all need," she says. Cognitive behavioral therapy assists us in stepping back in order to spot personal thought patterns that arise automatically and that we may want to move past.

A family therapist can also help sort through complicated sibling dynamics. Many parents feel guilty when the child with food allergies requires so much attention that the others don't get an equal share. Many siblings are protective of a brother or a sister with food allergies, which means they end up shouldering responsibilities that other children their age do not. Resentment could build over the fact that restaurants, vacations, and other family outings have to be shaped around keeping the food-allergic son or daughter safe. These dynamics can fester into unhealthy relationships over time if they aren't sorted out. Many siblings will be able to do this on their own as they mature. But working with a professional may help address certain issues sooner and ensure that concerns are fully dealt with.

IMMUNOTHERAPY ANXIETY

As we talked about above, the prospect of immunotherapy can carry its own set of anxieties because it involves eating a food that the body believes is a poison. Matthews emphasizes that the immunotherapy process is very different. The healthcare professional is not asking the peanut-allergic patient to suddenly eat a candy bar. "The experience of a carefully and rigorously designed food challenge is very different from an accidental exposure," notes Matthews, who works with families before, during, and after immunotherapy treatment. With immunotherapy, a patient consumes perhaps one one-hundredth of a peanut. The nurse or doctor is standing by. The treatment is in a healthcare facility. Simply explaining all of this to someone anxious about trying immunotherapy can go a long way toward alleviating the fear.

Here, the medical staff is often instrumental. Andy's mom, Kim, was grateful that Kari and her colleagues kept her son on track during his immunotherapy trial. When he put up a fuss, the physician was there to encourage him. "You're doing this," Kim recalls the physician telling her son. She didn't push him into something Andy didn't want to do, but she helped him find the strength to keep going when he was scared. Parents can't always play that role for their children. Because a doctor was there holding his hand and refusing to let go, Andy was ushered into a very different life than the one he would have lived without immunotherapy.

Recently, Alia Crum and our team conducted a study at Stanford to see if fostering an optimistic mind-set about immunotherapy could make the experience better. Along with their parents, we told fifty children, ages 7 to 17, who were going through peanut immunotherapy that the non-life-threatening symptoms of OIT were unfortunate side effects of the treatment (24 families) or that these symptoms signaled that desensitization was working (26 families). The families in the latter group were less anxious, less likely to inquire about symptoms with the staff, and less likely to skip doses. Curiously, the children in this group had fewer mild symptoms as the OIT dose increased, and their blood showed higher levels of IgG4, immune cells that signal a healthy response to a food protein.

We believe that not only are children with food allergy heroes but so are their families. One of the consequences of the medical history of this condition has been a poor recognition of just how much families go through. Living with a food allergy is like living with the constant threat of your home bursting into flames or a lion chasing you across the plains. On top of the fear are the many forms of emotional heartache that crop up over the years.

We urge families to seek help—from support groups, from friends, and above all, from one another. Denise Bunning, the cochair of MOCHA (Mothers of Children Having Allergies), a patient advocacy organization, emphasizes how much the food allergy world has changed since the mid-1990s, when she was raising children with the condition. "There is more awareness now and more options for accommodations." She also sees value in being able to give away your own hard-won wisdom. "Being able to share what works, as well as creative, positive solutions, with other families is extremely important," says Bunning, whose husband, David, cochairs FARE. In other words, the sense of isolation that food allergy may sometimes bring is also one of the easiest challenges to overcome. And addressing that aspect is often the snatch of the magician's scarf, where pulling on it leads to an abundance of healing. The appendix includes resources for finding networks locally and online. But when it comes to building a web of support, we also recommend the contact list in your phone.

THE BOTTOM LINE

- Food allergy can create stress and anxiety for the diagnosed individual and their family.

- People with food allergy should educate themselves and seek support groups and networks.

- As with any challenging situation, immunotherapy may churn up hidden stress within a family or an individual. Working with a therapist during this time may help.

CHOOSING YOUR PATH

Life changes when a person develops a food allergy, whether that happens soon after birth, as an adult, or any time between. The diagnosis changes your kitchen, your lifestyle, and the challenges you're destined to meet. We wrote this book so that people stepping into the world of food allergy for the first time—and those already entrenched—will have all the information they need to steer their own course. From infant diets to food labels, from prevention to treatment, from epinephrine to antibodies, the insights and studies described in these pages should give you all you need to know to keep you and your family not only safe but also thriving. Above all, we believe the compelling data on immunotherapy and the instructive how-to's for this treatment are information that everyone should have access to. It is our wish that in this new era, everyone with food allergy can live a life free from fear and compromise.

Tessa Grosso no longer lives with the multiple severe food allergies that plagued her childhood and sent her to the emergency room on several occasions. Immunotherapy retrained her immune system to welcome those former adversaries. Now she eats anything she wants. But as she explains, immunotherapy isn't about the taste of pizza. "Anyone who went through immunotherapy will say that eating the food is just a nice bonus," she says. "The true advantage is not having to worry."

But making it to the other side of food allergy transformed Tessa in an even deeper way. Now, as a teenager, she is speaking publicly about her experience to encourage others to take the reins of their own lives. "The only reason I have the life I do today is because my mom didn't just accept what the doctor told her," she says. She isn't advocating that people with food allergy don't listen to their physicians. Rather, she wants people to know that they are in control. "There could be something else out there for you, so you always have to look."

Tessa found that something else in immunotherapy. She found her way to a life where she doesn't have to live with the fear and anxiety that food allergy causes. Now Tessa wants to help others find their way there, too.

So do we. And we hope we are.

Chapter 11

THE FUTURE OF THE END OF FOOD ALLERGY

As this book has made clear, we believe that we are at the start of a very bright future for food allergy. Immunotherapy is offering powerful treatment options that free people from the fear of life-threatening allergic reactions. And our knowledge about how food allergies develop is teaching us how to prevent the condition from starting in the first place. That's why we called this book *The End of Food Allergy*—it is the end of an era founded on the mistaken belief that nothing can be done, and, we hope, the beginning of the end of food allergy, period.

Yet clinical advances aren't the only consideration as we look toward the future. We have to consider the rising rates of food allergy around the world. Countries where food allergies have not been a problem historically are now grappling with this new patient population. On the global scale, we are also facing the uncertainty of an environment rapidly undergoing disconcerting changes. Worsening food allergy is just one small consequence of the damage we've done to the planet.

Much can be done to counteract these troubling views of the future of food allergy. It may be cliché to say that small changes can make a big difference, but it's also true. To that end, we include some of these small steps here. We believe that those facing food allergy in the present could very well be the people to shape its future.

THE FUTURE OF THE FOOD ALLERGY POPULATION

Any view of the future for food allergy must take into account the fact that this is a global epidemic—increasingly so. Although the condition has been largely considered a Western world phenomenon, that scenario is rapidly changing. The rise of food allergy in Asia and Africa has led researchers to theorize that adopting a "Westernized" lifestyle may be contributing to food allergy diagnoses outside of North America and Europe. We don't yet have large amounts of evidence to support that idea, although researchers have observed spikes in food allergy rates among immigrants from non-Western countries who move to the United States, pointing to the role of diet and food preparation.

The lack of data makes accurate estimates difficult to come by. An oral food challenge is the gold standard for diagnosing the condition, but that test is too costly for many healthcare systems around the world. A study of food allergy prevalence in 89 countries found that only 9 had data based on oral food challenges and 51 had no relevant data at all. For 23 countries, awareness of food allergy rates depended mainly on parent reports of diagnoses or symptoms, a source that often leads to overestimating. Central and South America, Africa, Eastern Europe, and the Middle East are particularly underrepresented in the science so far. But the numbers we do have reveal one very clear truth: food allergy is a global disease.

Europe

Aware of rising food allergy rates, researchers from across Europe sought to measure the extent of the condition across the continent. Using local health registries in eight countries (Switzerland, Spain, the Netherlands, Poland, Bulgaria, Greece, Iceland, and Lithuania), they surveyed 240 people between the ages of 20 and 54 who had reported food allergy symptoms. About 4.4 percent of the individuals included in the survey had doctor-diagnosed food allergy, ranging from 1 percent in Vilnius, Lithuania, to 7.5 percent in Zurich, Switzerland. Nearly 19 percent of people from Madrid, Spain, said they'd reacted to at least one of the foods included in the survey, although not all had been diagnosed with food allergy.

The potential allergens the researchers inquired about included the familiar culprits in the United States, along with several fruits; vegetables and seeds; as well as lentils, mustard, and buckwheat. Following these initial responses, the researchers took blood samples from willing participants and also tested their homes for dust mites, pollen, and other airborne allergens. The researchers found IgE antibodies targeted against one or more food allergens in 24 percent of the participants from Zurich (the highest rate) and 7 percent in those from Reykjavík (the lowest rate). Sesame, shrimp, and hazelnut were the most common allergens; egg, milk, and fish were the most rare. Although the authors emphasize that having IgE specific to an allergen does not necessarily mean the person is actually allergic, the study contributes to the picture of food allergy rates across Europe.

Studies based on reports from parents and children in Slovenia, Estonia, Switzerland, Greece, and Belgium have reported food allergy rates of less than 5 percent. Others have found higher rates, such as one from Italy that reported food allergy in about 10 percent of children. A study in Sweden based on questionnaires about IgE levels and a history of allergic reactions found that about 3 percent of 1-year-olds and more than 7 percent of 8-year-olds had food allergy. In Germany, oral food challenges uncovered food allergies in 26 out of 739 children up to age 17, although rates in older children were lower than those among younger children. Although the most familiar food allergens in the United States are also the most problematic in Europe, apple and kiwi allergies are also common.

Africa

Studies in Ghana and South Africa have reported that about 5 percent of the population through their teenage years has food allergy, although that figure is based on IgE levels, which, again, don't always signify a food allergy, and skin prick tests, which can be faulty. When 400 households in Tanzania reported their experience of food allergy, researchers found rates as high as 17 percent (68 households). In a 2005 study in Mozambique, 97 of 509 people said they'd had some kind of food allergy at some point in their life, with many people reporting allergy to beef.

Asia

China has been paying attention to food allergy, as rates there have been rising. Starting in 2009, studies based on oral food challenges found prevalence rates in the southwestern region of the country between 3.8 percent and 7.7 percent, on par with many countries in Europe.

In Japan, Hong Kong, and Korea, studies based on reports from parents and children put the food allergy prevalence at about 5 percent. A survey based on questionnaires given to more than 30,000 people in Taiwan found that more than 3 percent of children under age 3, nearly 8 percent of children between the ages of 4 and 18, and more than 6 percent of adults had food allergy. Allergies to seafood were the most common type reported in that study.

A study in South India sought to separate food sensitivities from food allergy. Among 10,904 adults, at least 189 people reported some kind of reaction to a common allergen (hives, itchiness, vomiting, and other symptoms of food allergy). In a second part of the investigation, which included a more detailed survey and blood samples, the researchers found that about 1.2 percent of the 588 participants (7 people) probably had a true food allergy. Many more people—26.5 percent—said they were sensitive to at least one of the 24 foods the questionnaire inquired about, although as we've emphasized throughout this book, food sensitivity is not the same as food allergy.

South America

We don't have much data on food allergy rates in South America. In a survey of 3,099 children in Colombia, 10 percent of children up to age 8 and 12 percent of those between the ages of 9 and 16 said they were allergic to at least one food, although these rates are based on self-reports, which tend to be inflated. Fruit and vegetable allergies are common in Colombia, and so is allergy to meat.

Australia

Food allergy rates in Australia have escalated dramatically in recent years. A study from 2011 found that 280 out of 2,848 12-month-olds had a bona fide food allergy, confirmed by oral food challenge—a rate of 10 percent. This landmark study has led some experts to refer to Australia as "the food allergy capital of the world."

Middle East

The Middle East is another region without much data. A 2012 study asked Jewish and Arab adolescents in Israel about whether they had any history of food allergy. Among 11,171 completed questionnaires, the researchers found a prevalence rate of 3.6 percent (402 people). Peanut, egg, and sesame allergies were more common among Arab children, and milk allergy was more common among Jewish children. Supporting the theory of the atopic march—the procession from eczema to asthma to allergy that we see in many children—food allergy rates were higher among children with asthma in this study.

Summary

The 89-country study we mentioned at the start of this section provides persuasive evidence that food allergy is increasing in rapidly developing regions. The notion that Asian countries have lower rates of food allergy than European countries no longer holds true. Although we need more rigorous data for many regions of the world, these numbers already point to a new population of patients in need of treatments based on the most current research. And they make the continuing quest to understand the root causes of food allergy even more urgent.

THE FUTURE OF THE ENVIRONMENT

In light of what climate change portends—rising sea levels, crop-killing droughts, storms strong enough to flatten entire villages, temperature changes that will alter ecologies that have existed for millennia, and so much more—the link to food allergy may seem a small matter. But it's an under-recognized connection that could affect a huge portion of the global population. And considering that food allergy already costs an estimated $25 billion per year in just the United States alone, the possibility that global warming could worsen the epidemic is worth paying attention to.

Continued damage to the global environment will likely increase food allergy rates worldwide. "Climate change is affecting a host of diseases," says Marie Prunicki, MD, PhD, who studies the link between food allergy and the environment. "The whole allergen-asthma spectrum is impacted."

Changes to Allergenic Foods

For plants, rising temperatures spur adaptation. Trees, grass, flowers, and all other vegetation have to be able to withstand heat that they aren't accustomed to. For many species, that means playing defense. Plants need ways to protect themselves against heat. Just as we layer up in winter or slather sunscreen on in the summer, plants also have to adapt, but using only the equipment that lives inside their cells. And it turns out that some of the proteins that will allow plants to adapt to climate change are the same proteins that trigger food allergy. Research at Icahn School of Medicine at Mount Sinai has already shown that the amount of allergenic proteins can vary widely across a species; a peanut grown in Alabama faces different environmental stresses than a peanut grown in New Mexico, which could lead to different amounts of different proteins. Indeed, when scientists at the U.S. Department of Agriculture grew Virginia

Jumbo peanut plants in an environment with elevated levels of carbon dioxide, they produced greater concentrations of Ara h1, a protein strongly linked to peanut allergy, than the Georgia Green variety grown under the same conditions. And the theory is that the more the Ara h1 in a peanut, the higher the chance that the immune system will produce IgE antibodies against it.

In one of the first papers to chart the possible ties between climate change and food allergens, environmental scientists from Australia also noted that carbon dioxide and rising temperature may alter plants. Plants absorb this gas as part of photosynthesis, their process of turning sunlight into food. Heightened levels of carbon dioxide in the atmosphere may mean that plants don't need to invest as much energy in photosynthesis. That spare energy could be used in reproduction or storage, the researchers note. Many of the proteins that help protect the seeds inside a plant are also food allergens. Again, these changes may push allergenic protein levels up, which may make allergies likelier.

Changes to Pollen

Pollen is another slat on the bridge between climate change and food allergy. Temperature increases are extending pollen seasons. Pollen records from seventeen different locations in twelve countries show increases in recent years, stretching back to an average of 26 years. Warmer weather has been linked to a longer and more intense pollen season.

And pollen has a strong connection to food allergy. In a condition known as oral allergy syndrome, allergens found in pollen can trigger an immune reaction against raw fruits, vegetables, and some tree nuts. This particular form of allergy tends to arise in older children. The type of pollen allergy determines the type of food allergy—birch pollen is linked to allergies to apples and carrots (among others), whereas ragweed pollen is linked to allergies to banana and cucumber (among others). Cooking the food eliminates the allergic response because it alters the protein. You can see where all this is going: increased pollen counts mean increased amounts of allergenic protein, which means increased amounts of food allergy. Pollen sensitivities vary around the world, so the future could see regional differences in food allergy caused by oral allergy syndrome.

POLLEN AND FOOD CONNECTIONS IN ORAL ALLERGY SYNDROME	
THIS TYPE OF POLLEN . . .	MAY TRIGGER ALLERGIES TO . . .
Birch	Apple, apricot, cherry, peach, pear, plum, kiwi, carrot, celery, parsley, peanut, soybean, almond, hazelnut
Ragweed	Cantaloupe, honeydew, watermelon, zucchini, cucumber, banana, potato
Timothy and orchard grass	Peach, watermelon, orange, tomato, potato
Mugwort	Bell pepper, broccoli, cabbage, cauliflower, chard, garlic, onion, parsley, aniseed, caraway, coriander, fennel, black pepper

Rising temperatures are not the only environmental challenge we face. Pesticides, deforestation, a lack of crop diversity, a failure to rotate crops, pollution—all of this and more can affect the health of the soil, the air, the foods we eat, and our immune systems. They can also make plants more allergenic. In addition, modern lifestyles often limit the amount of time we spend in nature, reducing the number of microbes we're exposed to, which can also weaken immunity. The chemicals in our cleaning products and overly sanitized homes (as we spoke about in chapter 2) may do the same.

THE FUTURE OF LIVING WITH FOOD ALLERGIES

Throughout this book, at our Stanford clinic, and in all the conversations we have with food allergy families, there is one message we try to impart: you can take control. Food allergies can often leave a person feeling helpless. No matter how prepared you are, an allergen can sneak into a meal when you least expect it. The severity of a reaction can be equally unpredictable. Immunotherapy is, of course, a way to turn the tables on food allergy. But it isn't the only way. Simple lifestyle changes may help reduce the risk of developing food allergies. And there are ways to take action that may help the world become a safer place for people already living with the condition.

The Six Ds

There is a dual benefit to making lifestyle changes that favor environmentally friendly choices. Such measures reduce our impact on the environment and, as a by-product, may also reduce the risk of food allergy. Protecting the planet is the priority, and if doing so also makes food allergy less likely, then so much the better. Toward that end, we recommend following the Six Ds:

- **Detergent:** Many laundry detergents contain enzymes called proteases, which break down protein molecules. That makes these molecules effective stain removers, but it also makes them potentially unhealthy. Proteases may irritate the skin. Reports have linked proteases to dry skin and eczema, although the evidence behind this connection is mostly from animal studies, which are not reliable barometers for what might happen in humans. Researchers in Switzerland, led by the Akdis group, with Stanford have found that even at 1 part per billion (a very small amount), detergents can cause skin cells to break apart. Research is ongoing to better understand how detergents affect the skin and whether they contribute to the development of allergies.

  Harsh detergents are also bad for the enviroment. They create algae blooms in freshwater that deplete oxygen from the ecosystem, harming plants and fish. They also contain chemicals that can erode the mucous layers on the skin of fish that protect them from parasites, and also disrupt their endocrine system, leading to reproductive issues.

- **Dogs:** Although, again, the research is still in progress, many scientists suspect that our reduced exposure to a broad spectrum of microbes naturally present in nature may be compromising our immune systems. A pet dog is a perfect way to combat this depletion. Dogs are a vehicle for bringing nature inside your home. The dirt they track in after a walk and the mini-ecology that is their fur are likely to contain healthy bacteria that you may not otherwise be exposed to.

- **Diversity:** "Eat food. Not too much. Mostly plants," journalist and activist Michael Pollan famously began his book *In Defense of Food.* There are many reasons why these words are wise; one is because of the benefit of exposing ourselves to a wide range of the edible gifts nature has to offer. The more proteins and safe bacteria we expose our bodies to, the more vigorous our immune systems will become. As Dr. Sharon Chinthrajah, director of the clinical research unit at Stanford, often tells patients and families, keeping your diet diverse is an effective way to improve immunity and cultivate a healthy gut microbiome, which has a multitude of virtues.

- **Vitamin D:** Although studies have come to contradictory findings, we do have evidence of a link between vitamin D depletion and food allergy (as discussed in chapter 2). This link is another explanation for why modern lifestyles, which take place mostly indoors, may be at least partially responsible for the rise in food allergy. The sun spurs the production of vitamin D in our skin, and when we spend all our time indoors, that can't happen. Go outside. Let the sun shine on your skin. It will make you happy and it just may reduce your food allergy risk.

- **Dryness:** Dry skin raises the chance of developing eczema, which, as we've already discussed, raises the risk of food allergy. We recommend using moisturizer on dry skin to help prevent this situation. Helen Brough in the UK and others are working on identifying which moisturizers are best, because not all moisturizers are the same. We have found that wax- and petroleum-based products are not as effective as lipid-based products for treating dryness and reducing allergy risk. Steroid creams that decrease inflammation are safe for stubborn eczema and may help prevent allergies. Infants and children who maintain skin barrier protection using ceramide-based creams appear to develop fewer food allergies.

- **Dirt:** In line with many of the points above, spending less time outdoors, and getting dirty, may be compromising our immune systems. This is the thinking behind the hygiene hypothesis and the old friends hypothesis, as discussed in chapter 2. Again, the evidence wavers. We don't have solid proof that the reduced amount of time we spend in nature is responsible for the rise in food allergy. And we know that good hygiene practices save lives and must be followed (wash your hands!). But again, we have enough data to know that the range of microbes we encounter when we spend time outside dwarfs what we encounter in our homes. And we know that the gut microbiome is tied to immunity.

These personal changes are relatively simple. And even if the evidence is not yet conclusively in favor of them, they are also harmless. In cases like this, we adhere to the maxim "It can't hurt and it could help." But the effort to thwart food allergy doesn't stop at home. Rather, our homes are just the beginning.

FOOD ALLERGY POLICIES

Finally, we have to turn our attention to the policies and practices that shape our food system. The presence of food deserts—urban areas where access to fresh produce is extremely limited—contributes to health issues among people who are economically disadvantaged. Labeling laws fail to hold the makers of packaged foods to account. Restaurants are also often not held responsible for the presence of potentially fatal allergens even when a customer has asked about ingredients. Becoming active in local and state-based politics can be a powerful way to effect changes that make the world safer for those living with food allergy.

Several states now have laws related to food allergy awareness. In Illinois, restaurants must have a manager on duty who is trained in food allergy safety. The Massachusetts Department of Public Health now has an allergen awareness training program that issues a certificate upon completion for restaurants to display. A two-year effort by hundreds of people led to a Michigan law requiring food safety managers to receive food allergy awareness training. In Virginia, a food-allergic 14-year-old named Claire Troy presented her idea for a food allergy regulation to the state's house of delegates, which led to a law requiring the board of health to address food allergy in its training standards. These changes start with the individuals who are most affected by food allergy.

Other efforts have focused on ensuring epinephrine is available in public places. Many states now have laws allowing theme parks, sports venues, and other venues to keep epinephrine auto-injectors on hand for emergency use. Almost every state allows schools to stock undesignated epinephrine, and this trend is now reaching college campuses.

Food allergy activists are also fighting for better labeling laws.

After the hours that Kim and Dave Friedman spent trying to under-stand whether the food in their shopping cart was free from the risk of tree nut contamination (an odyssey we discussed in chapter 4), Kim has begun pushing for stricter regulations. "This is my life pas-sion now," she says. "It can be a matter of life and death for your child."

In short, there are countless ways for people with food allergy to become involved in fending off the creeping, invasive vines that con-tribute to the problem and help work toward better practices, better laws, and better awareness. The attention paid to food allergy is light-years beyond where it once was. Some relatives may never take it seriously. They may always continue to put out mixed nuts at the holidays. And even the most vigilant parents can never guaran-tee that their child won't accidentally encounter dairy or wheat or egg. But there is so much that families can now do, whether it's talk-ing about food allergy with a friend or taking the fight to your local city hall.

The new era of food allergy is all about empowerment. There is no reason to live in fear and isolation anymore. *The End of Food Allergy* is really just the beginning.

ACKNOWLEDGMENTS

FROM KARI

To my mentors, thank you for believing in me, teaching me, and taking the time to show me what I needed to see. To everyone who has participated in immunotherapy studies, thank you for your dedication and commitment. To all the patients who bravely carry the burden of food allergy, thank you for keeping us motivated to find better solutions. To the staff at the Sean N. Parker Center for Allergy & Asthma Research, thank you for the incredible care and attention you provide—and for sharing our vision. To Sean Parker, and other philanthropists, thank you for your incredible support.

To the National Institutes of Health; the FDA; the nonprofit organizations; Stanford, Lucile Packard Children's Hospital; Lucile Packard Foundation for Children's Health; the research institutions; the medical associations; the regulatory agencies; and the various companies involved in food allergy research, safety, and product development, thank you for delivering the innovations that can treat and prevent food allergy.

As much as food allergy research owes its progress to all these organizations, it owes just as much to the early believers. Many families who began with a vision of a life without allergies for their own children soon embraced a wider vision of helping to ensure all children would have access to the same advances. The pioneers are many. Thank you.

To my family and friends, thank you for supporting me every step of the way. There is no "my" before "accomplishments"; they are all ours together.

FROM SLOAN

Deepest thanks to Mary and Mark Weiser, who first told me at a wedding years ago about this remarkable doctor, right down the road from me, named Kari Nadeau, thereby setting my family on a course toward greater knowledge and healing. Thank you to Shannon Welch and J. R. Moehringer, who shepherded and championed this project in the early going. Enormous thanks to my three children, especially the two who endured the clinical trials for their food allergies. At the time we worried they were guinea pigs; now we know they were pioneers! And, of course, a million thanks to my husband, Roger, who shared with me those early fears and breathless questions about food allergies. His courage and patience and sage counsel have been invaluable in the course of my life, and in the making of this book.

FROM BOTH OF US

Thank you to our wonderful collaborator, acclaimed journalist Jessica Wapner, for her beautiful writing, skillful interviewing, and research; Caroline Sutton, editor extraordinaire at Penguin Random House, plus her crack team including Hannah Steigmeyer, Janice Kurzius, Linda Rosenberg, and copy editor Nancy Inglis; the fantastic Penguin Random House publicity and marketing crew, including Casey Maloney, Anne Kosmoski, Lindsay Gordon, and Farin Schlussel; visionary agents John Maas and Celeste Fine at Park & Fine Literary and Media; our brilliant lawyer Kim Schefler; Melanie Thernstrom for her thoughtful insights and for her interview notes; and the stellar Dr. Vanitha Sampath and Dr. Christopher Dant for their meticulous fact-checking and invaluable contributions to tables and figures.

Proceeds from book sales will be donated to nonprofit, nonacademic organizations focusing on research in food allergy.

APPENDIX 1: FOOD ALLERGY RESOURCES

Patient Advocacy and Support

Allergy & Asthma Network
For patients, families, and health professionals
www.aanma.org

AllergyHome
Organization dedicated to food allergy awareness and management
www.allergyhome.org

Allergy Ready
Online courses for families, educators, and anyone else involved in food
allergy care
www.allergyready.com

Asthma and Allergy Foundation of America
An organization for people living with asthma and allergy, and their
families
www.aafa.org

Food Allergy & Anaphylaxis Connection Team (FAACT)
Well-rounded resources for education and advocacy; runs one-week day
camps in three U.S. locations
www.foodallergyawareness.org

Kids with Food Allergies
A website and organization aimed at serving children living with food
allergies
www.kidswithfoodallergies.org

Mothers of Children Having Allergies (MOCHA)
Chicago-based nonprofit serving families with members who have
potentially life-threatening food allergy
www.mochallergies.org

SupportGroups.com: Food Allergy
Online forum for food allergy support
https://food-allergy.supportgroups.com

Key Government Agencies

Centers for Disease Control and Prevention (CDC)
www.cdc.gov

ClinicalTrials.gov
Database of federally funded clinical trials
www.clinicaltrials.gov

Immune Tolerance Network (ITN)
Research collaborative focused on developing immune tolerance
therapies and funded by the National Institutes of Health
www.immunetolerance.org

National Institute of Allergy and Infectious Diseases (NIAID)
www.niaid.nih.gov/diseases-conditions/food-allergy

U.S. Food and Drug Administration (FDA)
www.fda.gov

Safe Eating

Gluten Free Passport
A website that offers translation of phrases, travel checklists, and other
tips for traveling
https://glutenfreepassport.com

World Health Organization/International Union of Immunological
Societies (WHO/IUIS)
Allergen Nomenclature
Provides lists of scientific terminology related to various allergens
www.allergen.org

Nongovernment Organizations

End Allergies Together (EAT)
Funds research at several academic institutions across the United
States and hosts walkathons and other events
www.endallergiestogether.com

Food Allergy Research & Education (FARE)
Patient advocacy group that funds research and provides resources for
living with food allergies
www.foodallergy.org

Professional Medical Organizations

American Academy of Allergy, Asthma & Immunology (AAAAI)
www.aaaai.org

American Academy of Pediatrics (AAP)
www.aap.org

American College of Allergy, Asthma, & Immunology (ACAAI)
https://acaai.org

European Academy of Allergy and Clinical Immunology (EAACI)
www.eaaci.org

World Allergy Organization (WAO)
www.worldallergy.org

Magazines and Children's Books

Allergic Living magazine, www.allergicliving.com

Johansen, Alison Grace. *HumFree the Bee Has a Food Allergy*. Mascot Books, 2015.

Nelson, Ariella. *What's in this Cookie?* Hedgehog Graphics, 2019.

Recob, Amy. *The Bugabees: Friends with Food Allergies,* 2nd ed. Beaver's Pond Press, 2009.

Roderick, Christina. *No Peanuts for Pete*. Archway Publishing, 2016.

Santomero, Angela C. *Daniel Has an Allergy* (part of the Daniel Tiger's Neighborhood series). Simon Spotlight, 2017.

Skinner, Juniper. *Food Allergies and Me: A Children's Book*. CreateSpace Independent Publishing Platform, 2010.

Food Allergy Products for Children

A few of the many potentially useful products available online.

AllerMates
Medical charms, medical bags, epinephrine carrying cases, and other products for children with food allergy
https://allermates.com

FlatBox
Lunchboxes that convert into place mats
www.flatbox.com

Safety Tat
Allergy alert stickers
https://new.safetytat.com/product-category/medical-and-allergy/

StickyJ Medical
Medical alert bracelets (child size)
https://www.stickyj.com/category/medical-alert-id-bracelets-for-kids

Organizations Outside the United States

Swiss Institute of Allergy and Asthma Research (SIAF)
www.siaf.uzh.ch

Allergy & Anaphylaxis Australia
Nonprofit organization for allergy support
www.allergyfacts.org.au

Allergy New Zealand
National charity providing education, support, and information for
families with children who have allergies
www.allergy.org.nz

Food Allergy Canada
Resource for Canadian families living with food allergy
www.foodallergycanada.ca

Allergy UK
UK-based support for people living with allergic disease
www.allergyuk.org

Anaphylaxis Campaign
UK organization offering support groups, education, news, and training
specifically related to severe allergies
www.anaphylaxis.org.uk

Fundación S.O.S. Alergia
Patient advocacy group in Argentina
www.sosalergia.org

Allergy Care India
Membership-based nonprofit organization made up of pediatric and
adult food allergy patients and their families
www.allergycareindia.org

Epinephrine

Patient education: use of an epinephrine auto-injector (Beyond the
Basics)

www.uptodate.com/contents/use-of-an-epinephrine-autoinjector-beyond
-the-basics

Financial assistance
www.epipen.com/paying-for-epipen-and-generic

AUVI-Q home delivery service
www.auvi-q.com/pdf/Direct-Delivery-Service-Enrollment-Form.pdf

Other

Sean N. Parker Center for Allergy & Asthma Research at Stanford
University
Kari Nadeau, MD, PhD, director
www.med.stanford.edu/allergyandasthma/about-us.html

APPENDIX 2: DEBUNKING COMMON MYTHS

MYTH: It is unsafe to be vaccinated for influenza if you are allergic to eggs.

FACT: The influenza vaccine is safe for people with egg allergy; it does not activate the immune response to egg protein.

MYTH: Celiac disease is an allergy to wheat.

FACT: Celiac disease is not an allergy. It is a chronic immune disease but does not involve IgE antibodies, the hallmark of food allergy.

MYTH: People who are sensitive to gluten are allergic to wheat.

FACT: Gluten sensitivity is not a food allergy. It is also not the same as celiac disease. Diagnostic tests are available that can differentiate between these three conditions.

MYTH: All allergy tests are the same.

FACT: Some allergy tests are more effective—sometimes far more effective—than others. Be wary of tests that are not covered by insurance and must be paid for entirely out of pocket.

MYTH: Private allergy immunotherapy clinics are safe for treatment.

FACT: Not all of these clinics are the same. Be careful and ask critical questions before starting (see chapter 8 for a list of suggested questions).

MYTH: It's best to wait to introduce peanuts and other common allergens into a baby's diet.

FACT: Delayed introduction does not prevent food allergy and may actually increase the risk of food allergy.

MYTH: Your allergy will never change.

FACT: Allergic reactions can absolutely change over time. A mild reaction on one occasion does not predict a mild reaction next time. Reactions can transform from mild to severe, which means people with food allergy should always carry epinephrine.

APPENDIX 3: DISCLOSURES OF CONFLICT

The food allergy community is a tight-knit one. The shared goal of finding something better to offer patients has brought together researchers willing to do the work and families wanting to help in whatever way they can. Researchers also often have ties to pharmaceutical and other companies willing to take a chance on developing new treatments. They also often work with advocacy groups. As vital as we believe these ties to be, we feel it is equally vital to be transparent about them. Toward that end, we have included the following list of disclosures, so that readers will have the information.

Kari Nadeau: Kari has received grants from the National Institute of Allergy and Infectious Diseases (NIAID); Food Allergy Research & Education (FARE); End Allergies Together (EAT); AllerGenis; Ukko Pharma; the National Institute of Environmental Health Sciences (NIEHS); the National Heart, Lung, and Blood Institute (NHLBI); and the Environmental Protection Agency (EPA). She is involved in clinical trials funded in part or whole by Regeneron, Genentech, Aimmune Therapeutics, DBV Technologies, AnaptysBio, Adare Pharmaceuticals, and Stallergenes Greer. She receives research funding from Novartis, Sanofi, Astellas Pharma, and Nestlé. She is a member of the Data and Safety Monitoring Board at Novartis and NHLBI. She co-founded Before Brands (the multi-protein toddler snack discussed in chapter 9), Alladapt, Latitude (a private allergy clinic), and IgGenix. She is the chief intellectual officer at FARE and director of the World Allergy Organization (WAO) Center of Excellence at Stanford. She has received personal fees from Regeneron, AstraZeneca, ImmuneWorks, and COUR Pharmaceuticals. She is a consultant and advisory board member at Ukko Pharma, Before Brands, Alladapt, IgGenix, Probio, Vedanta, Centocor, Seed, Novartis, NHLBI, EPA, the National Scientific Committee of ITN, and

NIH Programs. She holds several U.S. patents related to food allergy (patent numbers 62/647,389; 62/119,014; 12/610,940; 12/686,121; 10/064,936; 62/767,444; application numbers S10-392).

Sloan Barnett: Board of directors of California Pacific Medical Center. Sloan's husband, Roger Barnett, is charmain and CEO of Shaklee Corporation, a leading health and wellness company.

Kim Yates: CEO of Latitude and FARE patient liaison

Kim and Alan Hartman: Co-chairs of FARE patient board, board chair of Latitude

David and Denise Bunning: David Bunning is the co-chair of FARE. Denise Bunning is the co-chair of MOCHA (Mothers of Children Having Allergies), a patient advocacy organization.

GLOSSARY

Adrenaline: Also known as epinephrine.

Albumin: Albumin is a protein. Those with egg allergy should avoid products with albumin, as egg whites contain albumin.

Allergic march: There is often a progression trend in allergic diseases that begins early in life. Infants are generally (but not always) first diagnosed with eczema, then food allergy, followed by allergic rhinitis and asthma. This natural progression of allergic diseases is called the allergic march.

Allergic rhinoconjunctivitis: Another term for hay fever.

Alpha gal allergy: This allergy is directed toward a carbohydrate (galactose-alpha-1,3-galactose) found in meats. Individuals with alpha gal allergy are allergic to certain meats.

Anaphylaxis: Anaphylaxis is a severe, potentially life-threatening allergic reaction that can occur within seconds to minutes of exposure to an allergen. In anaphylaxis, many organs are simultaneously affected.

Antibody: An antibody is a protein produced by cells as a defense against foreign substances. In allergy, certain foods are mistakenly thought to be harmful and the body produces an antibody called IgE to fight the invaders.

Antigens: In food allergy, an antigen is a food substance (generally protein in foods) that causes the allergic reaction.

Antihistamines: A drug that blocks the inflammatory actions of histamine.

Atopic dermatitis: Another term for eczema.

Atopic march: *See* allergic march.

Atopy: The predisposition to produce IgE on exposure to an allergen.

Basophil: Basophils are immune cells that store a number of different chemicals, such as histamine, which are released on interaction with an allergen and IgE and cause immediate allergic inflammatory reactions.

Biologic: A biologic is manufactured in a living system such as a microorganism, or a plant or animal cell. They are often produced using recombinant DNA technology.

Casein and caseinates: These are proteins found in mammalian milk. Those with milk allergy should avoid products with casein and caseinates.

Cochrane Review: Cochrane Reviews are systematic reviews and are internationally recognized as the highest standard in evidence-based healthcare.

Cytokines: Cytokines are produced by many types of immune cells. They act via cell receptors and are major players in immune responses to allergens. They can also regulate the maturation, growth, and responsiveness of particular cell populations. They can increase or decrease allergic reactions in complex ways.

Dendritic cells: Dendritic cells are found abundantly in barrier surfaces such as the skin, and act as immune sentinels. They are the first to recognize allergens and induce appropriate immune responses.

Desensitization: Treatment interventions that increase the amount of an allergen that a person is able to ingest without having an allergic reaction are said to desensitize the individual to the allergen. At the current time, it is thought that desensitization after treatment is lost after a period of time unless the allergen is ingested on a regular (daily or every other day) basis.

Double-blind, placebo-controlled food challenge (DBPCFC): A food challenge is the most definitive way of diagnosing a food allergy. In a DBPCFC, neither the doctor nor the patient knows if the patient is ingesting an allergen or a placebo, eliminating bias during ingestion of allergen and recording of symptoms.

Dual-allergen exposure theory: This theory suggests that exposure to food allergens through the skin can lead to allergy, while consumption of these foods at an early age may actually result in tolerance.

Endotoxin: Endotoxin is a component of the exterior cell wall of certain bacteria, such as *E. coli*.

Eosinophilic esophagitis (EoE): In EoE, immune cells called eosinophils are found in the esophagus, causing the esophagus to narrow. This is a type of food allergy, but it cannot be detected by measurement of IgE. It can often be resolved by eliminating the allergenic foods.

Epinephrine: Epinephrine acts quickly to reverse the effects of a severe allergic reaction by improving breathing, raising blood pressure, and reducing inflammation.

Filaggrin (FLG): A protein found in skin cells, which plays a crucial role in maintaining a healthy barrier and preventing exposure of the body to allergens via the skin.

Food intolerance: Food intolerance is not an allergic reaction and is not mediated by the immune system. It does not cause immediate life-threatening reactions. It could be due to toxins in foods, enzyme deficiencies, etc.

Food protein-induced enterocolitis syndrome (FPIES): A type of food allergy in infants and toddlers. However, it cannot be detected by measurement of IgE. Allergenic foods can cause vomiting, diarrhea, and dehydration. It generally resolves by the age of 5.

Food sensitivity: Some individuals may have high IgE levels (indicating an immune reaction) but do not react adversely on eating the foods. This is termed food sensitivity.

Gluten: Gluten is a mix of proteins found in wheat, rye, barley, and other grains.

Histamine: Histamine is a compound released by immune cells (mast cells and basophils) and is responsible for some of the symptoms of allergic reactions.

Hives: Hives are red, raised skin rashes that in allergic individuals are triggered by an allergen.

Human microbiome: The communities of bacteria, viruses, and fungi that live together on and inside the human body constitute the human microbiome.

Hygiene hypothesis: The hygiene hypothesis states that increased exposure to microorganisms, particularly in early childhood, contributes to the development of the immune system, leading to a decrease in autoimmune and allergic diseases.

Immune system: The immune system involves many types of cells, organs, proteins, and tissues, which are spread throughout the body. They protect the body against germs and other foreign invaders. In food allergy, the immune system mistakes the proteins in some foods as foreign invaders and attacks them.

Immunoglobulin E (IgE): IgE is an antibody found in high levels in those with allergy. It mediates allergic reactions.

Immunoglobulin G4 (IgG4): IgG4 is increased during immunotherapy for food allergies. It is thought to block the actions of IgE and to assist with desensitization.

Immunotherapy: Immunotherapy is a novel treatment for those with food allergies. Desensitization to the allergen that the person is allergic to is achieved by giving gradually increasing doses of the allergen. There are currently no standardized protocols and the treatment is mostly conducted in research centers or specialized allergy centers. Immunotherapy for food allergy can be via the oral, sublingual, or epicutaneous (through the skin) routes.

Lactose: Lactose is a sugar molecule found in milk. Some individuals lack an enzyme called lactase, which is necessary to digest the sugar. Those that lack the enzyme are lactose intolerant. Symptoms of lactose intolerance include stomach pain and bloating. It is not a food allergy.

Mast cells: Mast cells are immune cells that store a number of different chemicals, such as histamine, which are released on interaction with an allergen and IgE and cause immediate allergic inflammatory reactions.

Meta-analysis: Meta-analyses evaluate data from a number of different studies and therefore increase statistical power, making the conclusions stronger than those obtained from a single study.

Oral allergy syndrome (OAS): OAS is caused by cross-reacting proteins in foods and pollen and is therefore generally mild. The proteins that trigger a reaction to pollen also trigger a reaction to certain raw fruits and vegetables.

Prebiotics: Prebiotics are foods (primarily high-fiber foods) that feed the friendly bacteria in the gut and enhance gut health.

Single nucleotide polymorphisms (SNPs): An SNP represents differences in a single DNA building block (a nucleotide).

Sustained unresponsiveness: This is a measure of how long desensitization is maintained (without regular consumption of allergenic foods) after successful desensitization with therapy. Ideally, this is for the rest of one's life, and would then be termed *tolerance*. However, as follow-ups are hard to conduct long-term, researchers measure sustained unresponsiveness, which indicates how long one has maintained desensitization without consumption of regular foods.

T helper 1 (Th1): T helper 1 (Th1 cells) is a major subtype of T cells. Th1 cells are involved in suppressing immune allergic reactions.

T helper 2 (Th2): T helper 2 (Th2 cells) is a major subtype of T cells. Th2 cells increase allergic inflammatory reactions.

T regulatory cells (Tregs): T regulatory cells (Tregs) are a major subtype of T cells. They are involved in suppressing immune allergic reactions.

Tolerance: Tolerance is nonreactivity to common foods. Most of us are naturally tolerant of most foods throughout life. Being tolerant also indicates that one does not have to consume the foods on a regular basis to stay nonreactive to the foods.

Tree nuts: Allergies to tree nuts are common. Tree nuts include walnut, almond, hazelnut, cashew, pistachio, and Brazil nuts. They do not include allergenic foods such as peanuts (a legume) or seeds (sunflower, sesame).

Whey: Whey is a protein found in milk. Those with milk allergy should avoid products with whey.

NOTES

Chapter 1. Introducing the End of Food Allergy

13 More than 10 percent of American adults: Gupta RS, Warren CM, Smith BM, et al. Prevalence and severity of food allergies among US adults. *JAMA Netw Open.* 2019;2(1):e185630.

Chapter 2. The Food Allergy Epidemic: What Is Happening and Why

17 a high rate of false positives: Dunlop JH, Keet CA. Epidemiology of food allergy. *Immunol Allergy Clin North Am.* 2018;38(1):13–25.

17. The rate of egg allergy: Lack G. Update on risk factors for food allergy. *J Allergy Clin Immunol.* 2012;129(5):1187–97.

17   According to the most recent NHANES survey: McGowan EC, Keet CA. Prevalence of self-reported food allergy in the National Health and Nutrition Examination Survey (NHANES) 2007–2010. *J Allergy Clin Immunol.* 2013;132(5):1216–19.e1215.

18 A more recent study by researchers at Northwestern University: Gupta RS, Warren CM, Smith BM, et al. The public health impact of parent-reported childhood food allergies in the United States. *Pediatrics.* 2018;142(6).

18 a 2014 estimate put the prevalence among U.S. adults: Sicherer SH, Sampson HA. Food allergy: Epidemiology, pathogenesis, diagnosis, and treatment. *J Allergy Clin Immunol.* 2014;133(2):291–307; quiz 308.

18 A 2019 survey that we conducted with researchers at Northwestern: Gupta RS, Warren CM, Smith BM, et al. Prevalence and severity of food allergies among US adults. *JAMA Netw Open.* 2019;2(1):e185630.

18 In 2013, an international group of researchers led by the World Allergy Organization: Prescott SL, Pawankar R, Allen KJ, et al. A global survey of changing patterns of food allergy burden in children. *World Allergy Org J.* 2013;6(1):21.

20 shift has been well documented since the late 1990s: Lack G. Update on risk factors for food allergy. *J Allergy Clin Immunol.* 2012;129(5):1187–97.

20 Between 2009 and 2011, it increased another 5.1 percent: Centers for Disease Control and Prevention. *Trends in Allergic Conditions Among Children: United States, 1997–2011.* https://www.cdc.gov/nchs/products/databriefs/db121.htm.

20 Hospital visits for food allergy increased threefold: Lack G. Update on risk factors for food allergy. *J Allergy Clin Immunol.* 2012;129(5):1187–97.

20 In China, for example, food allergy among infants: Sicherer SH, Sampson HA. Food allergy: A review and update on epidemiology, pathogenesis, diagnosis, prevention, and management. *J Allergy Clin Immunol.* 2018;141(1):41–58.

20 107 out of every 1 million: Lack G. Update on risk factors for food allergy. *J Allergy Clin Immunol.* 2012;129(5):1187–97.

20 Back in 1997, less than half a percent of U.S. children: Sicherer SH, Munoz-Furlong A, Godbold JH, Sampson HA. US prevalence of self-reported peanut, tree nut, and sesame allergy: 11-year follow-up. *J Allergy Clin Immunol.* 2010;125(6):1322–26.

20 Over the next seven years, prevalence nearly doubled: Gupta RS, Warren CM, Smith BM, et al. The public health impact of parent-reported childhood food allergies in the United States. *Pediatrics.* 2018;142(6).

20 In one 2007 survey, 17 percent of respondents: Rona RJ, Keil T, Summers C, et al. The prevalence of food allergy: A meta-analysis. *J Allergy Clin Immunol.* 2007;120(3):638–46.

20–21 African American children were also at high risk of allergies: Mahdavinia M, Fox SR, Smith BM, et al. Racial differences in food allergy phenotype and health care utilization among US children. *J Allergy Clin Immunol Pract.* 2017;5(2):352–57.e351.

21 non-Hispanic black children: Centers for Disease Control and Prevention. *Trends in Allergic Conditions Among Children: United States, 1997–2011.* https://www.cdc.gov/nchs/products/databriefs/db121.htm.

22 most significant increase among Hispanic children: Lack G. Update on risk factors for food allergy. *J Allergy Clin Immunol.* 2012;129(5):1187–97.

22 "African ancestry was a notable risk factor": Ibid.

22 The exact immune mechanisms behind a food allergy: Ibid.

23 our immune systems remain weak: U.S. Food and Drug Administration. Asthma: The Hygiene Hypothesis. https://www.fda.gov/vaccines-blood-biologics/consumers-biologics/asthma-hygiene-hypothesis.

23 The use of bleach, antibacterial soap, and other cleansers: Scudellari M. News Feature: Cleaning up the hygiene hypothesis. *Proc Natl Acad Sci USA.* 2017;114(7):1433–36.

24 The more siblings, the lower the incidence: Karmaus W, Botezan C. Does a higher number of siblings protect against the development of allergy and asthma? A review. *J Epidemiol Community Health.* 2002;56(3):209–17.

24 family size and birth order were more strongly linked to hay fever: Strachan DP. Hay fever, hygiene, and household size. *BMJ.* 1989;299(6710):1259–60.

25 Children who attend day care during the first six months of life: Ball TM, Castro-Rodriguez JA, Griffith KA, et al. Siblings, day-care attendance, and the risk of asthma and wheezing during childhood. *N Engl J Med.* 2000;343(8):538–43.

25 All of the seventeen studies looking at hay fever incidence: Karmaus W, Botezan C. Does a higher number of siblings protect against the development of allergy and asthma? A review. *J Epidemiol Community Health.* 2002;56(3):209–17.

25 some infections activate a type of immune cell called T helper 1: Matricardi PM, Bonini S. High microbial turnover rate preventing atopy: a solution to inconsistencies impinging on the hygiene hypothesis? *Clin Exp Allergy*. 2000;30(11):1506–10.

25 an abundance of Th2 activity is: Scudellari M. News Feature: Cleaning up the hygiene hypothesis. *Proc Natl Acad Sci USA*. 2017;114(7):1433–36.

25 relatively cleaner air compared to urban areas like Munich: Wjst M. Another explanation for the low allergy rate in the rural Alpine foothills. *Clin Mol Allergy*. 2005;3:7; Wjst M, Reitmeir P, Dold S, et al. Road traffic and adverse effects on respiratory health in children. *BMJ*. 1993;307(6904):596–600.

26 endotoxin flips an essential switch: U.S. Food and Drug Administration. Asthma: The hygiene hypothesis. https://www.fda.gov/vaccines-blood-biologics /consumers-biologics/asthma-hygiene-hypothesis.

26 the molecule is plentiful in the natural environment: Williams LK, Ownby DR, Maliarik MJ, Johnson CC. The role of endotoxin and its receptors in allergic disease. *Ann Allergy Asthma Immunol*. 2005;94(3):323–32; U.S. Food and Drug Administration. Asthma: The hygiene hypothesis. https://www.fda .gov/vaccines-blood-biologics/consumers-biologics/asthma-hygiene-hypothesis.

26 contact with livestock: Riedler J, Eder W, Oberfeld G, Schreuer M. Austrian children living on a farm have less hay fever, asthma and allergic sensitization. *Clin Exp Allergy*. 2000;30(2):194–200.

26 the mattresses of the farm children had more endotoxin: von Mutius E, Braun-Fahrlander C, Schierl R, et al. Exposure to endotoxin or other bacterial components might protect against the development of atopy. *Clin Exp Allergy*. 2000;30(9):1230–34.

26 "Indoor endotoxin exposure early in life may protect": Gereda JE, Leung DY, Thatayatikom A, et al. Relation between house-dust endotoxin exposure, type 1 T-cell development, and allergen sensitisation in infants at high risk of asthma. *Lancet*. 2000;355(9216):1680–83.

26–27 allergies in Gabon: van den Biggelaar AH, van Ree R, Rodrigues LC, et al. Decreased atopy in children infected with Schistosoma haematobium: a role for parasite-induced interleukin-10. *Lancet*. 2000;356(9243):1723–27.

27 respiratory viruses . . . don't protect: Jolien S. Hello microbe my old friend: How a diverse microbiome trains the immune system against allergies. https://thedishonscience.stanford.edu/posts/microbe-old-friends-allergies/.

27 the link between endotoxin and allergy: Williams LK, Ownby DR, Maliarik MJ, Johnson CC. The role of endotoxin and its receptors in allergic disease. *Ann Allergy Asthma Immunol*. 2005;94(3):323–32.

28 This collection of "flora" influences: Mohajeri MH, Brummer RJM, Rastall RA, et al. The role of the microbiome for human health: from basic science to clinical applications. *Eur J Nutr*. 2018;57(Suppl 1):1–14.

28 The "old friends" theory: Rook GA, Martinelli R, Brunet LR. Innate immune responses to mycobacteria and the downregulation of atopic responses. *Curr Opin Allergy Clin Immunol.* 2003;3(5):337–42.

28 Fewer microbes make for an incomplete immune education: Jolien S. Hello microbe my old friend: How a diverse microbiome trains the immune system against allergies. https://thedishonscience.stanford.edu/posts /microbe-old-friends-allergies/.

29 a tie between a diverse microbiome: Ibid.

29 a powerful connection between a diverse diet and less asthma: Tsuang AJ, Nowak-Węgrzyn AH. Increased food diversity in the first year of life is inversely associated with allergic diseases. *Pediatrics.* 2014;134:S139—S140.

29 a lack of exposure to animals: Jolien S. Hello microbe my old friend: How a diverse microbiome trains the immune system against allergies. https:// thedishonscience.stanford.edu/posts/microbe-old-friends-allergies/.

29 University of Chicago food allergy researcher Cathy Nagler: Feehley T, Plunkett CH, Bao R, et al. Healthy infants harbor intestinal bacteria that protect against food allergy. *Nat Med.* 2019;25(3):448–53.

29 Talal Chatila at Boston Children's Hospital: Abdel-Gadir A, Stephen-Victor E, Gerber GK, et al. Microbiota therapy acts via a regulatory T cell MyD88/ RORgammat pathway to suppress food allergy. *Nat Med.* 2019;25(7):1164–74.

30 a very effective way to study the hygiene hypothesis: DIABIMMUNE. Welcome to the DIABIMMUNE Microbiome Project. https://pubs.broadinstitute .org/diabimmune.

30 poor hygiene has caused, and continues to cause, untold suffering: Bloomfield SF, Rook GA, Scott EA, et al. Time to abandon the hygiene hypothesis: new perspectives on allergic disease, the human microbiome, infectious disease prevention and the role of targeted hygiene. *Perspect Public Health.* 2016;136(4):213–24.

31 The red, itchy skin: Mayo Clinic. Atopic dermatitis (eczema). https://www .mayoclinic.org/diseases-conditions/atopic-dermatitis-eczema/symptoms-causes /syc-20353273.

32 researchers in the UK note that the dual-exposure hypothesis: Lack G. Update on risk factors for food allergy. *J Allergy Clin Immunol.* 2012;129(5):1187–97.

32 mice with injured skin had expanded and activated mast cells: Leyva-Castillo JM, Galand C, Kam C, et al. Mechanical skin injury promotes food anaphylaxis by driving intestinal mast cell expansion. *Immunity.* 2019;50(5):1262–75.e1264.

33 Dutch researchers found immune cells: van Reijsen FC, Felius A, Wauters EA, et al. T-cell reactivity for a peanut-derived epitope in the skin of a young infant with atopic dermatitis. *J Allergy Clin Immunol.* 1998;101 (2 Pt 1):207–209.

33 children whose skin had been exposed to a little bit of peanut oil:
Lack G, Fox D, Northstone K, Golding J. Factors associated with the
development of peanut allergy in childhood. *N Engl J Med.* 2003;348(11):977–85.

33 32 percent of children who had used skin cream: Boussault P, Leaute-
Labreze C, Saubusse E, et al. Oat sensitization in children with atopic
dermatitis: prevalence, risks and associated factors. *Allergy.*
2007;62(11):1251–56.

**33 a direct connection between environmental exposure and peanut
allergy:** Fox AT, Sasieni P, du Toit G, et al. Household peanut consumption as a
risk factor for the development of peanut allergy. *J Allergy Clin Immunol.*
2009;123(2):417–23.

34 Areas with more epinephrine prescriptions: Camargo CA, Jr., Clark S,
Kaplan MS, et al. Regional differences in EpiPen prescriptions in the United
States: the potential role of vitamin D. *J Allergy Clin Immunol.* 2007;120(1):
131–36; Poole A, Song Y, Brown H, et al. Cellular and molecular mechanisms of
vitamin D in food allergy. *J Cell Mol Med.* 2018;22(7):3270–77.

**34 55 percent lower for those born in summer compared to other
seasons:** Ibid.

**34 children born in autumn and winter had higher rates of food
allergy:** Mullins RJ, Clark S, Katelaris C, et al. Season of birth and childhood
food allergy in Australia. *Pediatr Allergy Immunol.* 2011;22(6):583–89.

**34 One Australian study found a stark difference between infants with
low levels of vitamin D:** Allen KJ, Koplin JJ, Ponsonby AL, et al. Vitamin D
insufficiency is associated with challenge-proven food allergy in infants. *J
Allergy Clin Immunol.* 2013;131(4):1109–16, 1116.e1101–1106.

34 2.39 times more likely among people low in vitamin D: Poole A, Song
Y, Brown H, et al. Cellular and molecular mechanisms of vitamin D in food
allergy. *J Cell Mol Med.* 2018;22(7):3270–77.

34 mothers who take vitamin D during pregnancy: Nwaru BI, Ahonen S,
Kaila M, et al. Maternal diet during pregnancy and allergic sensitization in the
offspring by 5 yrs of age: a prospective cohort study. *Pediatr Allergy Immunol.*
2010;21(1 Pt 1):29–37.

35 Supplemental vitamin D is often given to infants: Centers for Disease
Control and Prevention. Vitamin D. https://www.cdc.gov/breastfeeding
/breastfeeding-special-circumstances/diet-and-micronutrients/vitamin-d.html.

35 by age 31, people who'd taken vitamin D supplements since infancy:
Poole A, Song Y, Brown H, et al. Cellular and molecular mechanisms of vitamin
D in food allergy. *J Cell Mol Med.* 2018;22(7):3270–77.

35 In 2016, a group of German researchers: Junge KM, Bauer T, Geissler S,
et al. Increased vitamin D levels at birth and in early infancy increase offspring
allergy risk—evidence for involvement of epigenetic mechanisms.
J Allergy Clin Immunol. 2016;137(2):610–13.

35 mothers with high vitamin D rates at birth: Weisse K, Winkler S, Hirche F, et al. Maternal and newborn vitamin D status and its impact on food allergy development in the German LINA cohort study. *Allergy.* 2013;68(2):220–28.

35 Vitamin D may change the composition of our gut microbiome: Poole A, Song Y, Brown H, et al. Cellular and molecular mechanisms of vitamin D in food allergy. *J Cell Mol Med.* 2018;22(7):3270–77.

36 IgE antibodies were discovered in the mid-1960s: World Allergy Organization. IgE in Clinical Allergy and Allergy Diagnosis. https://www .worldallergy.org/education-and-programs/education/allergic-disease-resource -center/professionals/ige-in-clinical-allergy-and-allergy-diagnosis.

36 immunologists Kimishige and Teruko Ishizaka found an unidentified antibody: Ribatti D. The discovery of immunoglobulin E. *Immunol Lett.* 2016;171:1–4.

36 The Ishizakas continued to study IgE: Platts-Mills TA, Heymann PW, Commins SP, Woodfolk JA. The discovery of IgE 50 years later. *Ann Allergy Asthma Immunol.* 2016;116(3):179–82.

37 That encounter coaxes the cells to release histamine: Galli SJ, Tsai M. IgE and mast cells in allergic disease. *Nat Med.* 2012;18(5): 693–704; British Society for Immunology. Mast Cells. https://www .immunology.org/public-information/bitesized-immunology/cells /mast-cells.

37 the proteins often share certain traits: Janeway CJ, Travers P, Walport M. *The Production of IgE.* New York: Garland Science, 2001.

37–38 Enzymes, a type of protein, seem especially adept at provoking Th2: Ibid.

38 A wide range of environmental allergens cause IgE responses: American Academy of Allergy, Asthma, and Immunology. Allergy Statistics. https://www.aaaai.org/about-aaaai/newsroom /allergy-statistics.

39 a few possible genes that may be food allergy risk factors: Hong X, Tsai HJ, Wang X. Genetics of food allergy. *Curr Opin Pediatr.* 2009;21(6):770–76.

41 about 100 tons of food in a lifetime: Crowe SE, Perdue MH. Gastrointestinal food hypersensitivity: basic mechanisms of pathophysiology. *Gastroenterology.* 1992;103(3):1075–95.

42 Up to 20 percent of Americans: Zopf Y, Baenkler HW, Silbermann A, et al. The differential diagnosis of food intolerance. *Dtsch Arztebl Int.* 2009;106(21):359–69.

42 inflammatory bowel disease or Crohn's disease: Crowe SE, Perdue MH. Gastrointestinal food hypersensitivity: basic mechanisms of pathophysiology. *Gastroenterology.* 1992;103(3):1075–95.

42 Some tests are more involved: Zopf Y, Baenkler HW, Silbermann A, et al. The differential diagnosis of food intolerance. *Dtsch Arztebl Int.* 2009;106(21):359–69; quiz 369–70.

Chapter 3. Is It My Fault? Escaping the Blame Game

45–46 10 percent of children with food allergy had no family history: Koplin JJ, Allen KJ, Gurrin LC, et al. The impact of family history of allergy on risk of food allergy: a population-based study of infants. *Int J Environ Res Public Health.* 2013;10(11):5364–77.

46 832 food-allergic children: Gupta RS, Singh AM, Walkner M, et al. Hygiene factors associated with childhood food allergy and asthma. *Allergy Asthma Proc.* 2016;37(6):e140—e146.

46 The genetic influence, the researchers concluded: Sicherer SH, Furlong TJ, Maes HH, et al. Genetics of peanut allergy: a twin study. *J Allergy Clin Immunol.* 2000;106(1 Pt 1):53–56.

46 "Asthma and allergic diseases of childhood are highly heritable": Ullemar V, Magnusson PK, Lundholm C, et al. Heritability and confirmation of genetic association studies for childhood asthma in twins. *Allergy.* 2016;71(2):230–38.

46 a parent or sibling with food allergy: Koplin JJ, Allen KJ, Gurrin LC, et al. The impact of family history of allergy on risk of food allergy: a population-based study of infants. *Int J Environ Res Public Health.* 2013;10(11):5364–77.

47 a family history of eczema and egg allergy: Tariq SM, Stevens M, Matthews S, et al. Cohort study of peanut and tree nut sensitisation by age of 4 years. *BMJ.* 1996;313(7056):514–17.

47 Having a mother or father with food allergy: Tsai HJ, Kumar R, Pongracic J, et al. Familial aggregation of food allergy and sensitization to food allergens: a family-based study. *Clin Exp Allergy.* 2009;39(1):101–109.

47 A second study of twins, this time of 826 pairs in rural China: Liu X, Zhang S, Tsai HJ, et al. Genetic and environmental contributions to allergen sensitization in a Chinese twin study. *Clin Exp Allergy.* 2009;39(7):991–98.

47 parents born in East Asia: Carter CA, Frischmeyer-Guerrerio PA. The genetics of food allergy. *Curr Allergy Asthma Rep.* 2018;18(1):2.

48 That rate isn't much higher: Gupta RS, Walkner MM, Greenhawt M, et al. Food allergy sensitization and presentation in siblings of food allergic children. *J Allergy Clin Immunol Pract.* 2016;4(5):956–62.

48 Mutations in a gene called filaggrin: Brown SJ, Asai Y, Cordell HJ, et al. Loss-of-function variants in the filaggrin gene are a significant risk factor for peanut allergy. *J Allergy Clin Immunol.* 2011;127(3):661–67.

48 Changes in a group of genes known as the human leukocyte antigen (HLA) system: Howell WM, Turner SJ, Hourihane JO, et al. HLA class II

DRB1, DQB1 and DPB1 genotypic associations with peanut allergy: evidence from a family-based and case-control study. *Clin Exp Allergy.* 1998;28(2):156–62.

48 Another study of nearly 2,800 parents and children in the United States: ScienceDaily. Genetic causes of children's food allergies. https://www .sciencedaily.com/releases/2017/10/171024110707.htm; Marenholz I, Grosche S, Kalb B, et al. Genome-wide association study identifies the SERPINB gene cluster as a susceptibility locus for food allergy. *Nat Commun.* 2017;8(1):1056.

48 1,500 children in both countries: Marenholz I, Grosche S, Kalb B, et al. Genome-wide association study identifies the SERPINB gene cluster as a susceptibility locus for food allergy. *Nat Commun.* 2017;8(1):1056.

51 a publication focused on infant formula and breastfeeding: American Academy of Pediatrics. Committee on Nutrition. Hypoallergenic infant formulas. *Pediatrics.* 2000;106(2 Pt 1):346–49.

51 allergies . . . were equally common in both groups: Falth-Magnusson K, Kjellman NI. Development of atopic disease in babies whose mothers were receiving exclusion diet during pregnancy—a randomized study. *J Allergy Clin Immunol.* 1987;80(6):868–75.

52 the levels of IgE antibodies in the cord blood following birth: Ibid.

52 Five years later, the researchers revisited the first study: Ibid.

52 In 1999, a small study from South Africa: Frank L, Marian A, Visser M, et al. Exposure to peanuts in utero and in infancy and the development of sensitization to peanut allergens in young children. *Pediatr Allergy Immunol.* 1999;10(1):27–32.

52 Eating peanuts during pregnancy: Hourihane JO, Dean TP, Warner JO. Peanut allergy in relation to heredity, maternal diet, and other atopic diseases: results of a questionnaire survey, skin prick testing, and food challenges. *BMJ.* 1996;313(7056):518–21.

52 a group of British researchers turned to a massive bank of data: Lack G, Fox D, Northstone K, Golding J. Factors associated with the development of peanut allergy in childhood. *N Engl J Med.* 2003;348(11):977–85.

53 no persuasive evidence in favor of eliminating potential allergens from the prenatal diet: Greer FR, Sicherer SH, Burks AW; American Academy of Pediatrics Committee on Nutrition; American Academy of Pediatrics Section on Allergy and Immunology. Effects of early nutritional interventions on the development of atopic disease in infants and children: The role of maternal dietary restriction, breastfeeding, timing of introduction of complementary foods, and hydrolyzed formulas. *Pediatrics.* 2008;121(1):183–91.

53 Among 140 infants with IgE antibodies to peanut: Sicherer SH, Wood RA, Stablein D, et al. Maternal consumption of peanut during pregnancy is associated with peanut sensitization in atopic infants. *J Allergy Clin Immunol.* 2010;126(6):1191–97.

53 five trials with a total of 952 participants: Kramer MS, Kakuma R. Maternal dietary antigen avoidance during pregnancy or lactation, or both, for preventing or treating atopic disease in the child. *Cochrane Database Syst Rev.* 2012(9):Cd000133.

54 The World Health Organization (WHO) recommends exclusive breastfeeding: World Health Organization. https://www.who.int/topics /breastfeeding/en/.

55 breastfeeding for at least four months: Greer FR, Sicherer SH, Burks AW. The effects of early nutritional interventions on the development of atopic disease in infants and children: The role of maternal dietary restriction, breastfeeding, hydrolyzed formulas, and timing of introduction of allergenic complementary foods. *Pediatrics.* 2019;143(4).

55 Avoiding some food allergens may help prevent eczema in children: Muraro A, Dreborg S, Halken S, et al. Dietary prevention of allergic diseases in infants and small children. Part III: Critical review of published peer-reviewed observational and interventional studies and final recommendations. *Pediatr Allergy Immunol.* 2004;15(4):291–307.

55 two studies with a total of 523 participants: Kramer MS, Kakuma R. Maternal dietary antigen avoidance during pregnancy or lactation, or both, for preventing or treating atopic disease in the child. *Cochrane Database Syst Rev.* 2012(9):Cd000133.

55 recommendations on breastfeeding and allergy that advised against such dietary changes: Greer FR, Sicherer SH, Burks AW. The effects of early nutritional interventions on the development of atopic disease in infants and children: The role of maternal dietary restriction, breastfeeding, hydrolyzed formulas, and timing of introduction of allergenic complementary foods. *Pediatrics.* 2019;143(4).

55 The European Academy of Allergy and Clinical Immunology (EAACI): Ibid.

55 the Australasian Society of Clinical Immunology and Allergy (ASCIA): Australasian Society of Clinical Immunology and Allergy. Infant feeding and allergy prevention guidelines. https://www.allergy.org.au/images /pcc/ASCIA_Guidelines_infant_feeding_and_allergy_prevention.pdf.

56 For parents feeding their newborns with formula, the most recent recommendation: Greer FR, Sicherer SH, Burks AW. The effects of early nutritional interventions on the development of atopic disease in infants and children: The role of maternal dietary restriction, breastfeeding, hydrolyzed formulas, and timing of introduction of allergenic complementary foods. *Pediatrics.* 2019;143(4).

56 A 2008 study from Australia found: Koplin J, Dharmage SC, Gurrin L, et al. Soy consumption is not a risk factor for peanut sensitization. *J Allergy Clin Immunol.* 2008;121(6):1455–59.

56 Another large Australian study, this one from 2016: Goldsmith AJ, Koplin JJ, Lowe AJ, et al. Formula and breast feeding in infant food allergy: A population-based study. *J Paediatr Child Health.* 2016;52(4):377–84.

56 researchers at the University of Memphis: American Academy of Allergy, Asthma, and Immunology. New study examines effects of breast feeding, pumping and formula food on early childhood food allergy. https://www.aaaai .org/about-aaaai/newsroom/news-releases/breast-feeding-food-allergy.

57 The number of babies born by cesarean section: Boerma T, Ronsmans C, Melesse DY, et al. Global epidemiology of use of and disparities in caesarean sections. *Lancet.* 2018;392(10155):1341–48.

57 food allergy was a minor issue: Renz-Polster H, David MR, Buist AS, et al. Caesarean section delivery and the risk of allergic disorders in childhood. *Clin Exp Allergy.* 2005;35(11):1466–72.

57 the link between childhood asthma, a risk factor for food allergy, and C-sections: Thavagnanam S, Fleming J, Bromley A, et al. A meta-analysis of the association between Caesarean section and childhood asthma. *Clin Exp Allergy.* 2008;38(4):629–33.

58 Another meta-analysis homed in on food allergy: Bager P, Wohlfahrt J, Westergaard T. Caesarean delivery and risk of atopy and allergic disease: meta-analyses. *Clin Exp Allergy.* 2008;38(4):634–42.

58 an increased incidence among children born by C-section. Koplin J, Allen K, Gurrin L, et al. Is caesarean delivery associated with sensitization to food allergens and IgE-mediated food allergy: a systematic review. *Pediatr Allergy Immunol.* 2008;19(8):682–87.

58 512 children from birth through 2 years of age: Kvenshagen B, Halvorsen R, Jacobsen M. Is there an increased frequency of food allergy in children delivered by caesarean section compared to those delivered vaginally? *Acta Paediatr.* 2009;98(2):324–27.

59 when certain bacteria colonize the gut microbiome, the risk of food allergy increases: Bjorksten B, Sepp E, Julge K, et al. Allergy development and the intestinal microflora during the first year of life. *J Allergy Clin Immunol.* 2001;108(4):516–20.

59 allergy rates were low in Estonia: Sepp E, Julge K, Vasar M, et al. Intestinal microflora of Estonian and Swedish infants. *Acta Paediatr.* 1997;86(9):956–61.

59 higher amounts of a bacterial species known as *Staphylococcus aureus*: Bjorksten B, Naaber P, Sepp E, Mikelsaar M. The intestinal microflora in allergic Estonian and Swedish 2-year-old children. *Clin Exp Allergy.* 1999;29(3):342–46.

59 *Clostridium difficile* bacteria existed in greater numbers: Bottcher MF, Nordin EK, Sandin A, et al. Microflora-associated characteristics in faeces from allergic and nonallergic infants. *Clin Exp Allergy.* 2000;30(11):1590–96.

59 a Finnish study probed even deeper: Kalliomaki M, Kirjavainen P, Eerola E, et al. Distinct patterns of neonatal gut microflora in infants in whom atopy was and was not developing. *J Allergy Clin Immunol.* 2001;107(1):129–134.

60 A major Dutch study from 2007 looking at 957 infants: Penders J, Thijs C, van den Brandt PA, et al. Gut microbiota composition and development of atopic manifestations in infancy: the KOALA Birth Cohort Study. *Gut.* 2007;56(5):661–67.

60 The exact mechanics driving the colonizing of a newborn's gut: Stinson LF, Payne MS, Keelan JA. A critical review of the bacterial baptism hypothesis and the impact of cesarean delivery on the infant microbiome. *Front Med (Lausanne).* 2018;5:135.

61 four specific types of bacteria that differed in the meconium of infants: Ardissone AN, de la Cruz DM, Davis-Richardson AG, et al. Meconium microbiome analysis identifies bacteria correlated with premature birth. *PLOS One.* 2014;9(3):e90784.

61 infants delivered vaginally had more diverse microbiomes: Shi YC, Guo H, Chen J, et al. Initial meconium microbiome in Chinese neonates delivered naturally or by cesarean section. *Sci Rep.* 2018;8(1):3255.

61 In one study of 98 infants, the 15 babies born via C-section: Backhed F, Roswall J, Peng Y, et al. Dynamics and stabilization of the human gut microbiome during the first year of life. *Cell Host Microbe.* 2015;17(5):690–703; Stinson LF, Payne MS, Keelan JA. A critical review of the bacterial baptism hypothesis and the impact of cesarean delivery on the infant microbiome. *Front Med (Lausanne).* 2018;5:135.

61 the stools of infants born by C-section: Sakwinska O, Foata F, Berger B, et al. Does the maternal vaginal microbiota play a role in seeding the microbiota of neonatal gut and nose? *Benef Microbes.* 2017;8(5):763–78.

61 gut microbiomes plentiful in bifidobacteria: O'Callaghan A, van Sinderen D. Bifidobacteria and their role as members of the human gut microbiota. *Front Microbiol.* 2016;7:925.

62 babies delivered by elective C-section: Azad MB, Konya T, Maughan H, et al. Gut microbiota of healthy Canadian infants: profiles by mode of delivery and infant diet at 4 months. *CMAJ.* 2013;185(5):385–94.

63 The American College of Obstetricians and Gynecologists has declared: Committee Opinion No. 725: Vaginal Seeding. *Obstet Gynecol.* 2017;130(5):e274—e278.

65 A 2001 Finnish study of 72 premature babies and 65 full-term babies: Siltanen M, Kajosaari M, Pohjavuori M, Savilahti E. Prematurity at birth reduces the long-term risk of atopy. *J Allergy Clin Immunol.* 2001;107(2):229–34.

65 **food allergy rates among 13,980 children born in 1995:** Liem JJ, Kozyrskyj AL, Huq SI, Becker AB. The risk of developing food allergy in premature or low-birth-weight children. *J Allergy Clin Immunol.* 2007;119(5):1203–209.

65 **A study by David Fleischer at the University of Colorado:** Fleischer DM, Conover-Walker MK, Christie L, et al. The natural progression of peanut allergy: Resolution and the possibility of recurrence. *J Allergy Clin Immunol.* 2003;112(1):183–89.

65 **Other studies have reported rates closer to 20 percent:** Dhar M. Can you outgrow your allergies? https://www.livescience.com/39257-outgrow-allergies -go-away.html.

65 **many children who are allergic to eggs early in life:** Ibid.

Chapter 4. What Happens Now? Food Labels, Kitchens, Schools, and Other Essentials

73 **The food allergy advocacy organization Food Allergy Research & Education (FARE):** Food Allergy Research and Education (FARE). Creating a food allergy safety zone at home. https://www.foodallergy.org/sites/default/files /migrated-files/file/home-food-safety.pdf.

74 **President Theodore Roosevelt passed the Pure Food and Drug Act:** Schlosser E. The man who pioneered food safety. https://www.nytimes.com/2018 /10/16/books/review/poison-squad-deborah-blum.html.

74 **The Food and Drug Administration (FDA) already existed:** U.S. Food and Drug Administration. When and why was FDA formed? https://www .fda.gov/about-fda/fda-basics/when-and-why-was-fda-formed.

74 **The Fair Packaging and Labeling Act:** Federal Trade Commission. Fair Packaging and Labeling Act. https://www.ftc.gov/enforcement/rules /rulemaking-regulatory-reform-proceedings/fair-packaging -labeling-act.

74 **The Nutrition Labeling and Education Act:** Nutrition Labeling and Education Act of 1990. Amendment. https://www.govinfo.gov/content/pkg /STATUTE-104/pdf/STATUTE-104-Pg2353.pdf.

74 **All allergens . . . should be voluntarily listed on labels:** Besnoff S. May contain: Allergen labeling regulations. https://scholarship.law.upenn.edu/cgi /viewcontent.cgi?article=9446&context=penn_law_review.

74 **Between September 1999 and March 2000:** U.S. Food and Drug Administration. Food allergies: When food becomes the enemy. http://lobby .la.psu.edu/_107th/108_Food_Allergen_Act/Agency_Activities/FDA/FDA _Consumer_July-August_2001.htm.

75 **a news report in *BMJ*:** Josefson D. FDA targets snack foods industry over allergens. *BMJ.* 2001;322:883.

75 **Milk protein in processed foods:** Kellymom.com. Hidden Dairy "Cheat Sheet." https://kellymom.com/store/freehandouts/hidden-dairy01.pdf.

75 **Not every family with an egg-allergic member would know to avoid albumin:** Gombas K, Anderson E. The challenge of food allergens: An update. *Food Safety Magazine,* October/November 2001. https://www .foodsafetymagazine.com/magazine-archive1/octobernovember-2001 /the-challenge-of-food-allergens-an-update/.

75 **a 2001 article in *FDA Consumer,* an FDA publication:** U.S. Food and Drug Administration. Food Allergies: When Food Becomes the Enemy. http:// lobby.la.psu.edu/_107th/108_Food_Allergen_Act/Agency_Activities/FDA/FDA _Consumer_July-August_2001.htm.

75 **the Food Allergen Labeling and Consumer Protection Act of 2004:** U.S. Food and Drug Administration. Food Allergen Labeling and Consumer Protection Act of 2004 Questions and Answers. https://www.fda.gov/food /food-allergensgluten-free-guidance-documents-regulatory-information/ food-allergen-labeling-and-consumer-protection-act-2004-questions-and-answers.

76 **Canada and many other countries require packaged food companies to disclose the sesame:** Gupta RS, Warren CM, Smith BM, et al. Prevalence and severity of food allergies among US adults. *JAMA Netw Open.* 2019;2(1):e185630.

76 **Less common but still concerning allergens:** Food Allergy Research & Education (FARE). Other food allergens. https://www.foodallergy.org/common -allergens/other-food-allergens.

76 **aren't regulated by the FDA:** Holistic Perspectives. The problem with food allergen labeling. https://holistic-perspectives.com/2018/01/28 /the-problem-with-food-allergen-labeling/.

77 **this *may contain* sentence:** Besnoff S. May contain: Allergen labeling regulations. https://scholarship.law.upenn.edu/cgi/viewcontent.cgi?article=9446& context=penn_law_review.

77 **Yet the FDA has no guidelines:** Ibid.

77 **As one legal review of FALCPA puts it:** Ibid.

78 **some people with food allergy react to highly refined oils:** U.S. Food and Drug Administration. Have food allergies? Read the label. https://www.fda .gov/consumers/consumer-updates/have-food-allergies-read-label.

78 **Tree nuts, crustaceans, and fish:** Carabin IG. Food allergies and FALCPA (1) 2004. http://burdockgroup.com/food-allergies-and-falcpa-1-2004/.

78 **the exemption clause leaves much room for error:** Luccioli S, Fasano J. Evaluating labeling exemptions for food allergens. *Food Safety Magazine,* October/November 2008, https://www.foodsafetymagazine.com/magazine-archive1 /octobernovember-2008/evaluating-labeling-exemptions-for-food-allergens/.

79 **as of July 2018, the FDA has received just eight notifications and four petitions:** U.S. Food and Drug Admistration. Inventory of Notifications Received under 21 U.S.C. 343(w)(7) for Exemptions from Food Allergen Labeling. https:// www.fda.gov/food/food-labeling-nutrition/inventory-notifications-received-under -21-usc-343w7-exemptions-food-allergen-labeling.

79 a requirement for companies to create a "food allergen control plan": Besnoff S. May contain: Allergen labeling regulations. https://scholarship .law.upenn.edu/cgi/viewcontent.cgi?article=9446&context=penn_law_review.

79 In 2014, the European Union passed a new law: European Commission. Food information to consumers—legislation. https://ec.europa.eu /food/safety/labelling_nutrition/labelling_legislation_en.

79 Canada, by contrast: Food Standards Australia New Zealand. Plain English Allergen Labelling (PEAL). http://www.foodstandards.gov.au/code /proposals/Documents/P1044%20CFS.pdf.

79 the MMR (measles, mumps, rubella) and influenza vaccines: Food Allergy Research & Education (FARE). Egg Allergy and Vaccines. https://www .foodallergy.org/life-with-food-allergies/living-well-everyday/egg-allergy -and-vaccines.

79 Medications contained in gel caps: Land MH, Piehl MD, Burks AW. Near fatal anaphylaxis from orally administered gelatin capsule. *J Allergy Clin Immunol Pract.* 2013;1(1):99–100.

80 The term, which means "without protection" in Greek: Healthline. The long, strange history of the EpiPen. https://www.healthline.com/health -news/strange-history-of-epipen#1.

80 Back in 1859, a British doctor named Henry Salter: Arthur G. Epinephrine: a short history. *Lancet Respir Med.* 2015;3(5):350–51.

81 Eustachius, an Italian considered a founder of the science of human anatomy: Pearce JMS. Links between nerves and glands: The story of adrenaline. https://pdfs.semanticscholar.org/8a42/dca930f51a dae916568014b3abe4d4b5c81e.pdf.

81 "The effect upon the blood vessels": Ibid.

81 Within a few years, Jokichi Takamine: Ramsey L. The strange history of the EpiPen, the device developed by the military that turned into a billion- dollar business and now faces generic competition between Mylan and Teva. https://www.businessinsider.com/the-history-of-the-epipen-and-epinephrine -2016-8; Healthline. The long, strange history of the EpiPen. https://www .healthline.com/health-news/strange-history-of-epipen#1; Yamashima T. Jokichi Takamine (1854–1922), the samurai chemist, and his work on adrenaline. *J Med Biogr.* 2003;11(2):95–102.

81 epinephrine was once used to treat bubonic plague and bedwetting: Healthline. The long, strange history of the EpiPen. https://www .healthline.com/health-news/strange-history-of-epipen#1; Pearce JMS. Links between nerves and glands: The story of adrenaline. https://pdfs .semanticscholar.org/8a42/dca930f51adae916568014b3abe4d4b5c81e.pdf.

82 Our pupils dilate, our heart rate increases: Wikipedia. Adrenergic receptor. https://en.wikipedia.org/wiki/Adrenergic_receptor.

82 relaxing the smooth muscle lining the airways and raising blood pressure: Kemp SF, Lockey RF, Simons FE. Epinephrine: the drug of choice for anaphylaxis—a statement of the World Allergy Organization. *World Allergy Org J.* 2008;1(7 Suppl):S18—S26.

82 the drug also widens the airways: Ibid.

82 When a self-injector was invented in the 1970s: Bowden ME. A Mighty Pen. https://www.sciencehistory.org/distillations/a-mighty-pen.

82 The FDA approved the first brand-name product, the EpiPen, in 1987. Ramsey L. The strange history of the EpiPen, the device developed by the military that turned into a billion-dollar business and now faces generic competition between Mylan and Teva. https://www.businessinsider.com /the-history-of-the-epipen-and-epinephrine-2016-8.

82 Epinephrine is the drug of choice: Kemp SF, Lockey RF, Simons FE. Epinephrine: the drug of choice for anaphylaxis—a statement of the World Allergy Organization. *World Allergy Org J.* 2008;1(7 Suppl):S18—S26.

84 According to a study of 48 food fatalities in the UK between 1999 and 2006: Ibid.

84 three of every four people who've died from food anaphylaxis: Pumphrey R. Anaphylaxis: can we tell who is at risk of a fatal reaction? *Curr Opin Allergy Clin Immunol.* 2004;4(4):285–90.

84 Most deaths due to anaphylaxis occur: Kemp SF, Lockey RF, Simons FE. Epinephrine: the drug of choice for anaphylaxis—a statement of the World Allergy Organization. *World Allergy Org J.* 2008;1(7 Suppl):S18—S26.

84 And in a review of sixty-three U.S. deaths due to food anaphylaxis: Ibid.

84 pharmacies provide written instructions: Barnett CW. Need for community pharmacist-provided food-allergy education and auto-injectable epinephrine training. *J Am Pharm Assoc (2003).* 2005;45(4):479–85.

84 But even though most parents say they feel confident about using the injector: Arkwright PD, Farragher AJ. Factors determining the ability of parents to effectively administer intramuscular adrenaline to food allergic children. *Pediatr Allergy Immunol.* 2006;17(3):227–29.

84 In a 2006 review of 601 cases of anaphylaxis in the United States: Webb LM, Lieberman P. Anaphylaxis: a review of 601 cases. *Ann Allergy Asthma Immunol.* 2006;97(1):39–43.

84 One survey found that in nearly half of sixty-eight cases of food-related anaphylaxis: Kemp SF, Lockey RF, Wolf BL, Lieberman P. Anaphylaxis. A review of 266 cases. *Arch Intern Med.* 1995;155(16):1749–54.

85 A 2006 study found that for 122 UK children with food allergy: Arkwright PD, Farragher AJ. Factors determining the ability of parents to effectively administer intramuscular adrenaline to food allergic children. *Pediatr Allergy Immunol.* 2006;17(3):227–29.

85 A U.S. survey of 1,000 adults who'd had a severe anaphylactic reaction: Wood RA, Camargo CA, Jr., Lieberman P, et al. Anaphylaxis in

America: the prevalence and characteristics of anaphylaxis in the United States. *J Allergy Clin Immunol.* 2014;133(2):461–67.

85 they fail to encourage families to seek training: Pumphrey R. When should self-injectible epinephrine be prescribed for food allergy and when should it be used? *Curr Opin Allergy Clin Immunol.* 2008;8(3):254–60.

85 Having seen it demonstrated beforehand: Arkwright PD, Farragher AJ. Factors determining the ability of parents to effectively administer intramuscular adrenaline to food allergic children. *Pediatr Allergy Immunol.* 2006;17(3):227–29.

85 A study from 2016 looking at anxiety and quality of life among food allergy families: Fedele DA, McQuaid EL, Faino A, et al. Patterns of adaptation to children's food allergies. *Allergy.* 2016;71(4):505–13.

85 in a Montreal-based study of more than 1,200 children: Altman A, Wood RA. A majority of parents of children with peanut allergy fear using the epinephrine auto-injector. *Pediatrics.* 2014;134(Suppl 3):S148.

86 "Autoinjectors cannot save lives": Pumphrey R. When should self-injectible epinephrine be prescribed for food allergy and when should it be used? *Curr Opin Allergy Clin Immunol.* 2008;8(3):254–60.

86 More serious reactions should trigger immediate epinephrine use: Anagnostou K, Turner PJ. Myths, facts and controversies in the diagnosis and management of anaphylaxis. *Arch Dis Child.* 2019;104(1):83–90.

90 schools typically require that any auto-injectors have a shelf life of one year: Food Allergy Research & Education (FARE). Managing food allergies in the school setting: Guidance for parents. https://www.foodallergy.org /sites/default/files/migrated-files/file/school-parent-guide.pdf.

90 In 2016, Mylan, the pharmaceutical company selling the brand name EpiPen: Beard D. Drugmaker wants billions from Mylan related to EpiPen rival. http://wvmetronews.com/2019/08/14/drugmaker-wants -billions-from-mylan-related-to-epipen-rival/.

91 The hike left the company with about $1.1 billion in profits: Bakewell S. The troubled history of Mylan, founded by two U.S. Army buddies. https://www .bloomberg.com/news/articles/2019-07-27/the-troubled-history-of-mylan -founded-by-two-u-s-army-buddies; Mole B. Years after Mylan's epic EpiPen price hikes, it finally gets a generic rival. https://arstechnica.com/science /2018/08/fda-approves-generic-version-of-mylans-600-epipens-but-the-price -is-tbd/.

91 In August 2018, generic epinephrine finally became available: Healio. Epinephrine cost, education remain crucial obstacles in school health. https:// www.healio.com/pediatrics/allergy-asthma-immunology/news/print /infectious-diseases-in-children/%7B97c4b55e-bff8-4684-b72f-faa24e86fbea%7D /epinephrine-cost-education-remain-crucial-obstacles-in-school-health; U.S. Federal Drug Administration. FDA approves first generic version of EpiPen. https://www.fda.gov/news-events/press-announcements/fda-approves-first -generic-version-epipen.

91 the initial generic price tag was $300: Kokosky G. Newly approved generic version of EpiPen is not cheaper than available option. https://www .pharmacytimes.com/publications/issue/2019/january2019/newly-approved -generic-version-of-epipen-is-not-cheaper-than-available-option.

91 A new Illinois law requires insurance companies to cover epinephrine: Slachta A. Illinois becomes 1st state to mandate EpiPen coverage for kids. https://www.cardiovascularbusiness.com/topics/healthcare-economics /illinois-1st-state-mandate-epipen-coverage-kids.

91 Meanwhile, another auto-injector: Rubenfire A. EpiPen rival AUVI-Q to return to market; company promises affordability. https://www .modernhealthcare.com/article/20161026/NEWS/161029942 /epipen-rival-auvi-q-to-return-to-market-company-promises-affordability.

91 AUVI-Q is a smaller device: Kodjak A. An alternative to the EpiPen is coming back to drugstores. https://www.npr.org/sections/health-shots /2016/10/26/499425541/-alternative-to-the-epipen-is-coming-back-to-drugstores.

92 In a 2012 study of more than 500 food-allergic preschool children: Fleischer DM, Perry TT, Atkins D, et al. Allergic reactions to foods in preschool-aged children in a prospective observational food allergy study. *Pediatrics.* 2012;130(1):e25–e32.

93 consensus guidelines that educators across the country can follow: Allergy & Anaphylaxis Australia. School Resources. https://allergyfacts.org.au /allergy-management/schooling-childcare/school-resources; Food Allergy Canada. National school policies. https://foodallergycanada.ca/professional-resources /educators/school-k-to-12/national-school-policies/.

94 a small clinical trial with 68 people: Wang J, Jones SM, Pongracic JA, et al. Safety, clinical, and immunologic efficacy of a Chinese herbal medicine (Food Allergy Herbal Formula-2) for food allergy. *J Allergy Clin Immunol.* 2015;136(4):962–970.e961.

94 herbal formulas intended to ameliorate eczema, food allergy, and asthma: Gagné C. Dr. Li and her chinese herbal remedies. https://www .allergicliving.com/2015/12/15/dr-li-and-her-chinese-herbal-remedies/.

Chapter 5. The Avoidance Myth: What We Used to Think
99 a 13-year-old boy with an extreme reaction to eggs: Gospel Hall, Biography 89. Dr. Alfred T. Schofield. http://gospelhall .org/index.php/bible-teaching/138-history/brethren-biographies /3058-biography-89-dr-alfred-t-schofield.

99 The street had about a hundred doctor's offices: Wikipedia. Harley Street. https://en.wikipedia.org/wiki/Harley_Street.

99 his parents told Harley Street physician Alfred Schofield: Schofield AT. A case of egg poisonong. *Lancet.* 1908;1908:716.

99 in December of 1906: Smith M. Another person's poison. *Lancet.* 2014;384(9959):2019–20.

100 Titus Lucretius Cato: Cohen SG. The allergy archives: pioneers and milestones. https://www.jacionline.org/article/S0091-6749(08)00777-X/pdf.

101 A study in 1930 found: Ibid.

101 Moses Maimonides, a twelfth-century rabbi and physician: Thiara G, Goldman RD. Milk consumption and mucus production in children with asthma. *Can Fam Physician*. 2012;58(2):165–66.

101 avoiding peaches, apricots, and cucumbers: Rosner F. Moses Maimonides' treatise on asthma. *Thorax*. 1981;36(4):245–51.

101 And Richard III, king of England: Licence A. Was the downfall of Richard III caused by a strawberry? https://www.newstatesman.com/ideas/2013/08/was-downfall-richard-iii-caused-strawberry; Rosenkek J. Gesundheit. http://www.doctorsreview.com/history/mar06-history/.

101 In another, from 1929, a woman's finger turned red: Cohen SG. The allergy archives: pioneers and milestones. https://www.jacionline.org/article/S0091-6749(08)00777-X/pdf.

101 The word *allergy* first appeared in 1906: Igea JM. The history of the idea of allergy. *Allergy*. 2013;68(8):966–73.

101 Von Pirquet suspected a link between allergy and the immune system: Smith M. Another person's poison. *Lancet*. 2014;384(9959):2019–20.

102 the word *reaction* didn't seem to cut it: Turk JL. Von Pirquet, allergy and infectious diseases: a review. *J R Soc Med*. 1987;80(1):31–33.

102 *Allergy*, as Von Pirquet defined it: Ibid.

102 (The word comes from the Greek *allos*, meaning "other"): Lal A, Sunaina Waghray S, Nand Kishore NN. Skin prick testing and immunotherapy in nasobronchial allergy: our experience. *Indian J Otolaryngol Head Neck Surg*. 2011;63(2):132–35.

102 a way to test people for tuberculosis: Turk JL. Von Pirquet, allergy and infectious diseases: a review. *J R Soc Med*. 1987;80(1):31–33.

102 In 1912, a pediatrician named Oscar Schloss: Wuthrich B. History of food allergy. *Chem Immunol Allergy*. 2014;100:109–19.

103 An estimated 50 percent or more of skin prick tests: Food Allergy Research & Education (FARE). Skin Prick Tests. https://www.foodallergy.org/life-with-food-allergies/food-allergy-101/diagnosis-testing/skin-prick-tests.

103 "food allergists": Smith M. Another person's poison. *Lancet*. 2014;384(9959):2019–20.

103 In 1921, a 1-year-old baby nearly died: Ibid.

104 an allergist from California named Albert Rowe: Nigg JT, Holton K. Restriction and elimination diets in ADHD treatment. *Child Adolesc Psychiatr Clin N Am*. 2014;23(4):937–53; Rowe AH. Elimination diets and the patient's allergies; A handbook of allergy. *J Allergy Clin Immunol*. 1944;13(1):104.

104 diagnosing a food allergy through an elimination diet: Fagen H. Elimination diets: Medical & dietary detective work. https://nursingclio.org/2017 /04/12/elimination-diets-medical-dietary-detective-work/#footnoteref3; Smith M. Another person's poison. *Lancet.* 2014;384(9959):2019–20.

104 a session on a psychiatrist's couch would be the best treatment: Smith M. Another person's poison. *Lancet.* 2014;384(9959):2019–20.

105 Those who remained dedicated to food allergy: Ibid.

105 A 1989 report on seven worldwide deaths due to peanut allergy: Settipane GA. Anaphylactic deaths in asthmatic patients. *Allergy Proc.* 1989;10(4):271–74; Waggoner MR. Parsing the peanut panic: the social life of a contested food allergy epidemic. *Soc Sci Med.* 2013;90:49–55.

105 "Peanut allergy is the most worrisome food allergy issue": Schwartz RH. Allergy, intolerance, and other adverse reactions to foods. https://www .healio.com/pediatrics/journals/pedann/1992-10-21-10/%7B0c5b78db-f463-4260 -a4ca-2d2917149911%7D/allergy-intolerance-and-other-adverse-reactions-to-foods.

105 A 1999 report estimated that 1.1 percent of the U.S. population (3 million people) was allergic to peanuts: Sicherer SH, Munoz-Furlong A, Burks AW, Sampson HA. Prevalence of peanut and tree nut allergy in the US determined by a random digit dial telephone survey. *J Allergy Clin Immunol.* 1999;103(4):559–62.

105–6 "Desensitization does not work": Waggoner MR. Parsing the peanut panic: the social life of a contested food allergy epidemic. *Soc Sci Med.* 2013;90:49–55; Speer F. Food allergy: the 10 common offenders. *Am Fam Physician.* 1976;13(2):106–12.

106 Back in 1934, two pediatricians from Chicago: Grulee CG, Sanford HN. The influence of breast and artificial feeding on infantile eczema. *J Pediatrics.* 1936;9:223–25.

106 In the mid-1980s, a study in mice: Strobel S, Ferguson A. Immune responses to fed protein antigens in mice. 3. Systemic tolerance or priming is related to age at which antigen is first encountered. *Pediatr Res.* 1984;18(7):588–94.

106 In 1989, a group from California: Zeiger RS, Heller S, Mellon MH, et al. Effect of combined maternal and infant food-allergen avoidance on development of atopy in early infancy: a randomized study. *J Allergy Clin Immunol.* 1989;84(1):72–89.

107 infants who had no milk during their first six months: Hattevig G, Kjellman B, Sigurs N, et al. Effect of maternal avoidance of eggs, milk, and fish during lactation upon allergic manifestations in infants. *Clin Exp Allergy.* 1989;19(1):27–32.

107 In 2003, a German study of 945 infants: von Berg A, Koletzko S, Grubl A, et al. The effect of hydrolyzed milk formula for allergy prevention in the first year of life: the German Infant Nutritional Intervention Study, a randomized double-blind trial. *J Allergy Clin Immunol.* 2003;111(3):533–40.

107 Beginning in 1998, UK health authorities suggested: Committee on Toxicity of Chemicals in Food, Consumer Products and the Environment: Peanut Allergy. https://webarchive.nationalarchives.gov.uk/20120403140904/http://cot .food.gov.uk/pdfs/cotpeanutall.pdf.

107 The American Academy of Pediatrics (AAP) followed suit starting in 2000: American Academy of Pediatrics. Committee on Nutrition. Hypoallergenic infant formulas. *Pediatrics.* 2000;106(2 Pt 1):346–49; Perkin MR, Logan K, Tseng A, et al. Randomized trial of introduction of allergenic foods in breast-fed infants. *N Engl J Med.* 2016;374(18):1733–43.

107 In 2003, the AAP and two pediatric medical societies in Europe published guidelines: Zeiger RS. Food allergen avoidance in the prevention of food allergy in infants and children. *Pediatrics.* 2003;111(6 Pt 3):1662–71.

108 By 2008, however, most pediatric authorities in most countries recommended: Agostoni C, Decsi T, Fewtrell M, et al. Complementary feeding: a commentary by the ESPGHAN Committee on Nutrition. *J Pediatr Gastroenterol Nutr.* 2008;46(1):99–110.

108 Allergists at Mount Sinai and Duke University: Maloney JM, Sampson HA, Sicherer SH, Burks WA. Food allergy and the introduction of solid foods to infants: a consensus document. *Ann Allergy Asthma Immunol.* 2006;97(4):559–60; author reply 561–52.

108 The European Society for Paediatric Gastroenterology, Hepatology and Nutrition: Agostoni C, Decsi T, Fewtrell M, et al. Complementary feeding: a commentary by the ESPGHAN Committee on Nutrition. *J Pediatr Gastroenterol Nutr.* 2008;46(1):99–110.

108 New parents often delayed the introduction of solid foods: Agostoni C, Decsi T, Fewtrell M, et al. Complementary feeding: a commentary by the ESPGHAN Committee on Nutrition. *J Pediatr Gastroenterol Nutr.* 2008;46(1):99–110.

108 20 percent of German mothers were postponing the introduction of solid foods: Ibid.

108 researchers in the UK reported in 2016: Du Toit G, Foong RX, Lack G. Prevention of food allergy—Early dietary interventions. *Allergol Int.* 2016;65(4):370–77.

109 What did the scientific research really show about avoidance?: de Silva D, Geromi M, Halken S, et al. Primary prevention of food allergy in children and adults: Systematic review. *Allergy.* 2014;69(5):581–89.

110 The SPACE (Study on the Prevention of Allergy in Children in Europe) trial: Halmerbauer G, Gartner C, Schier M, et al. Study on the prevention of allergy in Children in Europe (SPACE): allergic sensitization in children at 1 year of age in a controlled trial of allergen avoidance from birth. *Pediatr Allergy Immunol.* 2002;13(s15):47–54.

110 **And a 2007 study of 120 infants on the Isle of Wight:** Arshad SH, Bateman B, Sadeghnejad A, et al. Prevention of allergic disease during childhood by allergen avoidance: the Isle of Wight prevention study. *J Allergy Clin Immunol.* 2007;119(2):307–13.

110 **A handful of other studies in the seventy-four-study review showed a similar trend:** Halken S, Host A, Hansen LG, Osterballe O. Effect of an allergy prevention programme on incidence of atopic symptoms in infancy. A prospective study of 159 "high-risk" infants. *Allergy.* 1992;47(5):545–53; Bardare M, Vaccari A, Allievi E, et al. Influence of dietary manipulation on incidence of atopic disease in infants at risk. *Ann Allergy.* 1993;71(4):366–71; Marini A, Agosti M, Motta G, Mosca F. Effects of a dietary and environmental prevention programme on the incidence of allergic symptoms in high atopic risk infants: three years' follow-up. *Acta Paediatr Suppl.* 1996;414:1–21; Bruno G, Milita O, Ferrara M, et al. Prevention of atopic diseases in high risk babies (long-term follow-up). *Allergy Proc.* 1993;14(3):181–86; discussion 186–87; de Silva D, Geromi M, Halken S, et al. Primary prevention of food allergy in children and adults: Systematic review. *Allergy.* 2014;69(5):581–89.

110 **In 2010, the National Institute of Allergy and Infectious Diseases (NIAID):** Boyce JA, Assa'ad A, Burks AW, et al. Guidelines for the Diagnosis and Management of Food Allergy in the United States: Summary of the NIAID-Sponsored Expert Panel Report. *J Allergy Clin Immunol.* 2010;126(6):1105–18.

111 **In 2012, a committee with the American Academy of Allergy, Asthma, and Immunology:** Fleischer DM, Spergel JM, Assa'ad AH, Pongracic JA. Primary prevention of allergic disease through nutritional interventions. *J Allergy Clin Immunol Pract.* 2013;1(1):29–36.

111 **avoiding dust mites, pollen, or pet dander:** Boyce JA, Assa'ad A, Burks AW, et al. Guidelines for the Diagnosis and Management of Food Allergy in the United States: Summary of the NIAID-Sponsored Expert Panel Report. *J Allergy Clin Immunol.* 2010;126(6):1105–18.

113 **researchers from the UK and Portugal reported in 2013:** Brough HA, Santos AF, Makinson K, et al. Peanut protein in household dust is related to household peanut consumption and is biologically active. *J Allergy Clin Immunol.* 2013;132(3):630–38.

113 **Peanut residue lingers for three hours:** Brough HA, Makinson K, Penagos M, et al. Distribution of peanut protein in the home environment. *J Allergy Clin Immunol.* 2013;132(3):623–29.

113 **exposure through their skin:** Brough HA, Liu AH, Sicherer S, et al. Atopic dermatitis increases the effect of exposure to peanut antigen in dust on peanut sensitization and likely peanut allergy. *J Allergy Clin Immunol.* 2015;135(1):164–70.

115 **In the past, complaints of food-triggered reactions:** May CD. Are confusion and controversy about food hypersensitivity really necessary? *J Allergy Clin Immunol.* 1985;75(3):329–33.

115 sociologists have raised concerns that hype surrounding peanut allergy: Waggoner MR. Parsing the peanut panic: the social life of a contested food allergy epidemic. *Soc Sci Med.* 2013;90:49–55.

116 Plenty of other medical conditions: Sampson HA. Food allergy. Part 2: diagnosis and management. *J Allergy Clin Immunol.* 1999;103(6):981–89.

117 A diary can reveal a source of contamination: Ibid.

118 Skin prick tests pose very little risk: Pitsios C, Dimitriou A, Stefanaki EC, Kontou-Fili K. Anaphylaxis during skin testing with food allergens in children. *Eur J Pediatr.* 2010;169(5):613–15.

118 the high rate of false positives: Boyce JA, Assa'ad A, Burks AW, et al. Guidelines for the Diagnosis and Management of Food Allergy in the United States: Summary of the NIAID-Sponsored Expert Panel Report. *J Allergy Clin Immunol.* 2010;126(6):1105–18.

118 Skin prick tests are less than 50 percent accurate: Sampson HA. Food allergy. Part 2: diagnosis and management. *J Allergy Clin Immunol.* 1999;103(6):981–89.

118 False negatives are extremely rare: Ibid.

118 babies under 2 years of age are particularly prone to having smaller wheals: Ibid.

118 a false-positive rate of 50 percent or more: Food Allergy Research and Education (FARE). Blood Tests. https://www.foodallergy.org/life-with-food -allergies/food-allergy-101/diagnosis-testing/blood-tests.

118 Blood tests can be costly: Sicherer SH, Wood RA. Allergy testing in childhood: using allergen-specific IgE tests. *Pediatrics.* 2012;129(1):193–97.

119 a person with peanut allergy may test positive for a grass pollen allergy: Food Allergy Research & Education (FARE). Blood Tests. https://www .foodallergy.org/life-with-food-allergies/food-allergy-101/diagnosis-testing /blood-tests.

120 the oral food challenge: Sampson HA. Immunologically mediated food allergy: the importance of food challenge procedures. *Ann Allergy.* 1988;60(3):262–69.

120 Verified in the early 1980s as the gold standard for diagnosing food allergy: Bernstein M, Day JH, Welsh A. Double-blind food challenge in the diagnosis of food sensitivity in the adult. *J Allergy Clin Immunol.* 1982;70(3):205–10.

121 Peanut challenges may start with the equivalent of a tenth of a nut: Nowak-Wegrzyn A, Assa'ad AH, Bahna SL, et al. Work Group report: oral food challenge testing. *J Allergy Clin Immunol.* 2009;123(6 Suppl):S365—S383.

122 The first basophil activation tests (BATs) emerged a few years ago: MacGlashan DW, Jr. Basophil activation testing. *J Allergy Clin Immunol.* 2013;132(4):777–87; McGowan EC, Saini S. Update on the performance and

application of basophil activation tests. *Curr Allergy Asthma Rep.*
2013;13(1):101–109.

122 The tests measure the extent to which the basophils: McGowan EC,
Saini S. Update on the performance and application of basophil activation tests.
Curr Allergy Asthma Rep. 2013;13(1):101–109.

Chapter 6. Turning the Tables: The Science—and How-Tos—of Early Introduction

125 he had seen the disturbing data: Hourihane JO, Aiken R, Briggs R,
et al. The impact of government advice to pregnant mothers regarding peanut
avoidance on the prevalence of peanut allergy in United Kingdom children at
school entry. *J Allergy Clin Immunol.* 2007;119(5):1197–202.

126 a curious study from the Netherlands on nickel allergy: Van
Hoogstraten IM, Andersen KE, Von Blomberg BM, et al. Reduced frequency of
nickel allergy upon oral nickel contact at an early age. *Clin Exp Immunol.*
1991;85(3):441–45.

126 A 1996 study by researchers in Norway and Finland: Kerosuo H,
Kullaa A, Kerosuo E, et al. Nickel allergy in adolescents in relation to
orthodontic treatment and piercing of ears. *Am J Orthod Dentofacial Orthop.*
1996;109(2):148–54.

126 Maybe that was just how the body worked: Du Toit G, Katz Y,
Sasieni P, et al. Early consumption of peanuts in infancy is associated with a low
prevalence of peanut allergy. *J Allergy Clin Immunol.* 2008;122(5):984–91.

127 Lack knew the evidence: Lack G, Fox D, Northstone K, Golding J.
Factors associated with the development of peanut allergy in childhood.
N Engl J Med. 2003;348(11):977–85.

127 Lotions to treat eczema that contained peanut oil: Ibid.

**127 infants with peanut allergy were exposed to peanuts through their
environment:** Fox AT, Lack G. High environmental exposure to peanut in
infancy as a risk factor for peanut allergy. *J Allergy Clin Immunol.*
2005;115(2):S34.

127 Bits of egg, milk, and fish: Du Toit G, Katz Y, Sasieni P, et al. Early
consumption of peanuts in infancy is associated with a low prevalence of peanut
allergy. *J Allergy Clin Immunol.* 2008;122(5):984–91.

**127 wheat allergy was more common among infants who hadn't eaten
cereal until after 6 months of age:** Poole JA, Barriga K, Leung DY, et al.
Timing of initial exposure to cereal grains and the risk of wheat allergy.
Pediatrics. 2006;117(6):2175–82.

**127 lower rates of asthma, eczema, and allergic rhinitis (more
commonly known as hay fever):** Asher MI, Montefort S, Bjorksten B, et al.
Worldwide time trends in the prevalence of symptoms of asthma, allergic
rhinoconjunctivitis, and eczema in childhood: ISAAC Phases One and Three
repeat multicountry cross-sectional surveys. *Lancet.* 2006;368(9537):733–43.

128 And both countries had high levels of asthma: Du Toit G, Katz Y, Sasieni P, et al. Early consumption of peanuts in infancy is associated with a low prevalence of peanut allergy. *J Allergy Clin Immunol.* 2008;122(5):984–91.

128 Lack and his team knew the implications of their results: Ibid.

129 Learning Early About Peanut Allergy (LEAP): Du Toit G, Roberts G, Sayre PH, et al. Randomized trial of peanut consumption in infants at risk for peanut allergy. *N Engl J Med.* 2015;372(9):803–13.

132 a consensus statement that recommended early introduction of peanut to high-risk infants: Fleischer DM, Sicherer S, Greenhawt M, et al. Consensus communication on early peanut introduction and the prevention of peanut allergy in high-risk infants. *Pediatrics.* 2015;136(3): 600–604.

132 Hugh Sampson, a pediatric allergist at Mount Sinai Hospital in New York: Kim M. The new wisdom on nut allergies and infants: Pediatricians endorse early exposure. https://www.washingtonpost.com/news /to-your-health/wp/2015/10/01/the-new-wisdom-on-nut-allergies-and-infants -pediatricians-endorse-early-exposure/.

132 The results, published in *The New England Journal of Medicine* in 2016: Du Toit G, Sayre PH, Roberts G, et al. Effect of avoidance on peanut allergy after early peanut consumption. *N Engl J Med.* 2016;374(15):1435–43.

133 Another study, known as Enquiring About Tolerance (EAT): Perkin MR, Logan K, Marrs T, et al. Enquiring About Tolerance (EAT) study: Feasibility of an early allergenic food introduction regimen. *J Allergy Clin Immunol.* 2016;137(5):1477–86.e1478.

133 Just like the American Academy of Pediatrics, this panel: Togias A, Cooper SF, Acebal ML, et al. Addendum guidelines for the prevention of peanut allergy in the United States: Report of the NIAID-Sponsored Expert Panel. https://www.niaid.nih.gov/sites/default/files/addendum-peanut-allergy -prevention-guidelines.pdf; Togias A, Cooper SF, Acebal ML, et al. Addendum guidelines for the prevention of peanut allergy in the United States: Report of the National Institute of Allergy and Infectious Diseases-sponsored expert panel. *Ann Allergy Asthma Immunol.* 2017;118(2):166–73.e167.

135 A Japanese study called Prevention of Egg Allergy with Tiny Amounts (PETIT): Natsume O, Kabashima S, Nakazato J, et al. Two-step egg introduction for prevention of egg allergy in high-risk infants with eczema (PETIT): a randomised, double-blind, placebo-controlled trial. *Lancet.* 2017;389(10066):276–86.

135 In 2013, researchers from Australia and Sweden: Palmer DJ, Metcalfe J, Makrides M, et al. Early regular egg exposure in infants with eczema: A randomized controlled trial. *J Allergy Clin Immunol.* 2013;132(2): 387–92.e381.

136 The egg powder, it seemed, had reduced the development of allergy: Wei-Liang Tan J, Valerio C, Barnes EH, et al. A randomized trial of egg introduction from 4 months of age in infants at risk for egg allergy. *J Allergy Clin Immunol.* 2017;139(5):1621–28.e1628.

136 5.6 percent of the intervention group had egg sensitivity: Bellach J, Schwarz V, Ahrens B, et al. Randomized placebo-controlled trial of egg consumption for primary prevention in infants. *J Allergy Clin Immunol.* 2017;139(5):1591–99.e1592.

136 Five trials provided moderate-certainty evidence: Ierodiakonou D, Garcia-Larsen V, Logan A, et al. Timing of allergenic food introduction to the infant diet and risk of allergic or autoimmune disease: A systematic review and meta-analysis. *JAMA.* 2016;316(11):1181–92.

141 And it makes putting dinner on the table that much easier: Australasian Society of Clinical Immunology and Allergy. Infant feeding and allergy prevention guidelines. https://www.allergy.org.au/images/pcc/ASCIA _Guidelines_infant_feeding_and_allergy_prevention.pdf.

142 Study in Rural Environments . . . which included 856 children: Roduit C, Frei R, Depner M, et al. Increased food diversity in the first year of life is inversely associated with allergic diseases. *J Allergy Clin Immunol.* 2014;133(4):1056–64.

Chapter 7. Beyond Avoidance: The Brave New World of Immunotherapy

145 more than 60 million people around the world living with the disease: Food Allergy Research and Education (FARE). Facts and Statistics. https://www.foodallergy.org/life-with-food-allergies/food-allergy-101/facts-and -statistics.

148 History tells us that King Mithridates VI: Hyden M. Mithridates' poison elixir: Fact or fiction? https://www.ancient.eu/article/906 /mithridates-poison-elixir-fact-or-fiction/.

148 The practice of desensitizing people with respiratory allergies: OIT 101. History of OIT. https://www.oit101.org/history -of-oit/.

149 the slow introduction of tiny amounts of allergens: Wood RA. Oral immunotherapy for food allergy. *J Investig Allergol Clin Immunol.* 2017;27(3):151–59.

149 a notable increase in IgG4: Vickery BP, Lin J, Kulis M, et al. Peanut oral immunotherapy modifies IgE and IgG4 responses to major peanut allergens. *J Allergy Clin Immunol.* 2013;131(1):128–34 .e121–123; Sampath V, Sindher SB, Zhang W, Nadeau KC. New treatment directions in food allergy. *Ann Allergy Asthma Immunol.* 2018;120(3): 254–62.

149 IT also appears to increase the number of regulatory T cells: National Institutes of Health. NIH scientists find link between allergic and autoimmune diseases in mouse study. https://www.nih.gov/news-events

/news-releases/nih-scientists-find-link-between-allergic-autoimmune-diseases -mouse-study; Sampath V, Sindher SB, Zhang W, Nadeau KC. New treatment directions in food allergy. *Ann Allergy Asthma Immunol.* 2018;120(3):254–62.

149 IT also appears to decrease the amount of T helper type 2: Dominguez-Villar M, Hafler DA. Regulatory T cells in autoimmune disease. *Nat Immunol.* 2018;19(7):665–73; Sampath V, Sindher SB, Zhang W, Nadeau KC. New treatment directions in food allergy. *Ann Allergy Asthma Immunol.* 2018;120(3):254–62. Tomicic S, Falth-Magnusson K, Bottcher MF. Dysregulated Th1 and Th2 responses in food-allergic children—does elimination diet contribute to the dysregulation? *Pediatr Allergy Immunol.* 2010;21(4 Pt 1):649–55.

150 a desensitization treatment on nineteen people with a range of single food allergies: Patriarca C, Romano A, Venuti A, et al. Oral specific hyposensitization in the management of patients allergic to food. *Allergol Immunopathol (Madr).* 1984;12(4):275–81.

151 The first substantial trial came in the late 1990s: Nelson HS, Lahr J, Rule R, et al. Treatment of anaphylactic sensitivity to peanuts by immunotherapy with injections of aqueous peanut extract. *J Allergy Clin Immunol.* 1997;99(6 Pt 1):744–51.

151 The results, combined with the findings of a 1992 study of subcutaneous immunotherapy: Oppenheimer JJ, Nelson HS, Bock SA, et al. Treatment of peanut allergy with rush immunotherapy. *J Allergy Clin Immunol.* 1992;90(2):256–62.

152 Patriarca and his group returned to the medical literature in 1998: Patriarca G, Schiavino D, Nucera E, et al. Food allergy in children: results of a standardized protocol for oral desensitization. *Hepatogastroenterology.* 1998;45(19):52–58.

152 59 people with food allergy underwent oral desensitization: Patriarca G, Nucera E, Roncallo C, et al. Oral desensitizing treatment in food allergy: Clinical and immunological results. *Aliment Pharmacol Ther.* 2003;17(3):459–65.

152 The next significant step forward came from Germany: Staden U, Rolinck-Werninghaus C, Brewe F, et al. Specific oral tolerance induction in food allergy in children: efficacy and clinical patterns of reaction. *Allergy.* 2007;62(11):1261–69.

154 researchers at Johns Hopkins University, led by Robert Wood, randomized 20 children: Skripak JM, Nash SD, Rowley H, et al. A randomized, double-blind, placebo-controlled study of milk oral immunotherapy for milk allergy. *J Allergy Clin Immunol.* 2008;122(6): 1154–60.

155 Almost all of the sixty 2-year-old children in one study from Spain: Martorell A, De la Hoz B, Ibanez MD, et al. Oral desensitization as a useful treatment in 2-year-old children with milk allergy. *Clin Exp Allergy.* 2011;41(9):1297–1304.

155 a study of milk-allergic schoolchildren in Finland: Salmivesi S, Korppi M, Makela MJ, Paassilta M. Milk oral immunotherapy is effective in school-aged children. *Acta Paediatr.* 2013;102(2):172–76.

155 By the end of 2014, at least 278 milk-allergic children: Begin P, Chinthrajah RS, Nadeau KC. Oral immunotherapy for the treatment of food allergy. *Hum Vaccin Immunother.* 2014;10(8): 2295–302.

155 A group of researchers from Spain: Vazquez-Ortiz M, Alvaro-Lozano M, Alsina L, et al. Safety and predictors of adverse events during oral immunotherapy for milk allergy: Severity of reaction at oral challenge, specific IgE and prick test. *Clin Exp Allergy.* 2013;43(1):92–102.

155 In a 2007 study of 7 children, all the participants tolerated more egg protein: Buchanan AD, Green TD, Jones SM, et al. Egg oral immunotherapy in nonanaphylactic children with egg allergy. *J Allergy Clin Immunol.* 2007;119(1):199–205.

155 After a year, all 6 children could eat more than one egg with no reaction: Itoh N, Itagaki Y, Kurihara K. Rush specific oral tolerance induction in school-age children with severe egg allergy: one year follow up. *Allergol Int.* 2010;59(1):43–51.

155 A year later, a Spanish team reported their results: Garcia Rodriguez R, Urra JM, Feo-Brito F, et al. Oral rush desensitization to egg: efficacy and safety. *Clin Exp Allergy.* 2011;41(9):1289–96.

155 By 2014, of the 165 children who participated in egg OIT studies: Begin P, Chinthrajah RS, Nadeau KC. Oral immunotherapy for the treatment of food allergy. *Hum Vaccin Immunother.* 2014;10(8): 2295–302.

155 And in 2017, a group from France: Morisset M, Moneret-Vautrin DA, Guenard L, et al. Oral desensitization in children with milk and egg allergies obtains recovery in a significant proportion of cases. A randomized study in 60 children with milk allergy and 90 children with egg allergy. *Eur Ann Allergy Clin Immunol.* 2007;39(1):12–19.

156 4 children had their peanut allergy completely disappear: Clark AT, Islam S, King Y, et al. Successful oral tolerance induction in severe peanut allergy. *Allergy.* 2009;64(8):1218–20.

156 In Arkansas, 20 out of 28 enrolled children: Hofmann AM, Scurlock AM, Jones SM, et al. Safety of a peanut oral immunotherapy protocol in children with peanut allergy. *J Allergy Clin Immunol.* 2009;124(2):286–91, 291.e281–e286.

156 And 298 patients—85 percent—were able to tolerate: Wasserman RL, Factor JM, Baker JW, et al. Oral immunotherapy for peanut allergy: multipractice experience with epinephrine-treated reactions. *J Allergy Clin Immunol Pract.* 2014;2(1):91–96.

156 By the end of 2014, at least 516 peanut-allergic children: Begin P, Chinthrajah RS, Nadeau KC. Oral immunotherapy for the treatment of food allergy. *Hum Vaccin Immunother.* 2014;10(8):2295–302.

157 Among the most important of these trials was PALISADE: Vickery BP, Vereda A, Casale TB, et al. AR101 Oral Immunotherapy for Peanut Allergy. *N Engl J Med.* 2018;379(21):1991–2001.

158 Another bedrock study, known as POISED (Peanut Oral Immunotherapy Study: Safety, Efficacy, and Discovery): Chinthrajah RS, Purington N, Andorf S, et al. Sustained outcomes in oral immunotherapy for peanut allergy (POISED study): a large, randomised, double-blind, placebo-controlled, phase 2 study. *Lancet.* 2019;394(10207):1437–49.

158 After two years, 84 percent of the treatment group: Sampath V, Tupa D, Graham MT, et al. Deciphering the black box of food allergy mechanisms. *Ann Allergy Asthma Immunol.* 2017;118(1):21–27.

159 lower levels of IgE antibodies and other allergy indicators: Science Daily. Few people with peanut allergy tolerate peanut after stopping oral immunotherapy. https://www.sciencedaily.com/releases/2019/09 /190913120828.htm.

160 Donald Leung and colleagues had tried omalizumab: Leung DYM, Sampson HA, Yunginger JW, et al. Effect of anti-IgE therapy in patients with peanut allergy. *N Engl J Med.* 2003; 348; 986–93.

160 Eleven children who had a history of strong reactions to milk: Nadeau KC, Schneider LC, Hoyte L, et al. Rapid oral desensitization in combination with omalizumab therapy in patients with milk allergy. *J Allergy Clin Immunol.* 2011;127(6):1622–24.

161 the sooner a person is freed from allergies the better: Ibid.

161 Our second phase 1 study: Bégin P, Winterroth LC, Dominguez T, et al. Safety and feasability of oral immunotherapy to multiple allergens for food allergy. *Allergy Asthma Clin Immunol.* 2014; 10:1.

168 A *New York Times Magazine* story on OIT: Thernstrom M. The allergy buster. https://www.nytimes.com/2013/03/10/magazine/can-a-radical-new -treatment-save-children-with-severe-allergies.html.

168 In a phase 2 study at Stanford, we randomized 48 children: Andorf S, Purington N, Block WM, et al. Anti-IgE treatment with oral immunotherapy in multifood allergic participants: a double-blind, randomised, controlled trial. *Lancet Gastroenterol Hepatol.* 2018;3(2):85–94.

171 lives were improved emotionally and socially: Epstein-Rigbi N, Goldberg MR, Levy MB, et al. Quality of life of food-allergic patients before, during, and after oral immunotherapy. *J Allergy Clin Immunol Pract.* 2019;7(2): 429–36.e422.

171 A team of researchers in the UK measured quality of life: Anagnostou K, Islam S, King Y, et al. Study of induction of tolerance to oral peanut: a randomised controlled trial of desensitisation using peanut oral immunotherapy in children (STOP II). Efficacy and Mechanism Evaluation No. 1.4. Southampton (UK); 2014.

171 Multi-allergen immunotherapy studies around the world: Scurlock AM. Oral and sublingual immunotherapy for treatment of IgE-mediated food allergy. *Clin Rev Allergy Immunol.* 2018;55(2):139–52; Otani IM, Bégin P, Kearney C, et al. Multiple-allergen oral immunotherapy improves quality of life in caregivers of food-allergic pediatric subjects. *Allergy Asthma Clin Immunol.* 2014;10(1):25; Bégin P, Dominguez T, Wilson SP, et al. Phase 1 results of safety and tolerability in a rush oral immunotherapy protocol to multiple foods using Omalizumab. *Allergy Asthma Clin Immunol.* 2014;10(1):7.

171 more than 40 parents of children enrolled in an OIT study: Otani IM, Bégin P, Kearney C, et al. Multiple-allergen oral immunotherapy improves quality of life in caregivers of food-allergic pediatric subjects. *Allergy Asthma Clin Immunol.* 2014;10(1):25.

172 desensitization remained in former peanut OIT patients who didn't eat nuts for a full year: Chinthrajah RS, Purington N, Andorf S, et al. Sustained outcomes in oral immunotherapy for peanut allergy (POISED study): a large, randomised, double-blind, placebo-controlled, phase 2 study. *Lancet.* 2019;394(10207):1437–49.

175 In the early 2000s, a group in Spain: American College of Allergy Asthma and Clinical Immunology. Sublingual Immunotherapy (SLIT). https://acaai.org/allergies/allergy-treatment/allergy-immunotherapy/sublingual -immunotherapy-slit; Enrique E, Pineda F, Malek T, et al. Sublingual immunotherapy for hazelnut food allergy: a randomized, double-blind, placebo-controlled study with a standardized hazelnut extract. *J Allergy Clin Immunol.* 2005;116(5):1073–79.

176 In their 2013 report of the study, the researchers noted that a year of SLIT: Fleischer DM, Burks AW, Vickery BP, et al. Sublingual immunotherapy for peanut allergy: a randomized, double-blind, placebo-controlled multicenter trial. *J Allergy Clin Immunol.* 2013;131(1):119–27.e111–117.

176 The researchers, led by David Fleischer in Denver: Burks AW, Wood RA, Jones SM, et al. Sublingual immunotherapy for peanut allergy: Long-term follow-up of a randomized multicenter trial. *J Allergy Clin Immunol.* 2015;135(5):1240–48.e1241–43.

176 OIT was more effective for treating peanut allergy: Narisety SD, Frischmeyer-Guerrerio PA, Keet CA, et al. A randomized, double-blind, placebo-controlled pilot study of sublingual versus oral immunotherapy for the treatment of peanut allergy. *J Allergy Clin Immunol.* 2015;135(5):1275–82.e1271–76.

176 Ten patients reached the level of sustained unresponsiveness: Kim EH, Yang L, Ye P, et al. Long-term sublingual immunotherapy for peanut allergy in children: Clinical and immunologic evidence of desensitization. *J Allergy Clin Immunol.* 2019;144(5):1320–26.e1321.

177 A phase 1 study of 100 peanut-allergic people: Jones SM, Agbotounou WK, Fleischer DM, et al. Safety of epicutaneous immunotherapy for the treatment of peanut allergy: A phase 1 study using the Viaskin patch. *J Allergy Clin Immunol.* 2016;137(4):1258–61.e1210.

177 A phase 3 study soon followed: Jones SM, Sicherer SH, Burks AW, et al. Epicutaneous immunotherapy for the treatment of peanut allergy in children and young adults. *J Allergy Clin Immunol.* 2017;139(4):1242–52.e1249.

178 Researchers in North Carolina and Australia joined forces: Tang ML, Ponsonby AL, Orsini F, et al. Administration of a probiotic with peanut oral immunotherapy: A randomized trial. *J Allergy Clin Immunol.* 2015;135(3):737–44.e738.

178 Four years later, the researchers reported: Hsiao KC, Ponsonby AL, Axelrad C, et al. Long-term clinical and immunological effects of probiotic and peanut oral immunotherapy after treatment cessation: 4-year follow-up of a randomised, double-blind, placebo-controlled trial. *Lancet Child Adolesc Health.* 2017;1(2):97–105.

179 In 2017, the European Academy of Allergy and Clinical Immunology (EAACI) released: Europen Academy of Allergy and Clinical Immunology (EAACI). Allergen Immunotherapy Guidelines Part 2: Recommendations. https://www.eaaci.org/documents/Part_II_-_AIT_Guidelines_-_web_edition.pdf.

180 In 2019, the Australasian Society of Clinical Immunology and Allergy (ASCIA) advised: Australasian Society of Clinical Immunology and Allergy. Oral Immunotherapy for Food Allergy. https://www.allergy.org.au/patients/allergy-treatment/oral-immunotherapy-for-food-allergy.

180 "peanut OIT can be safe and effective": Wang J, Bird AJ. What you should know about immunotherapy for food allergies. https://www.aappublications.org/news/2019/05/31/oralimmunotherapy053119?sso=1&sso_redirect_count=1&nfstatus=401&nftoken=00000000-0000-0000-0000-000000000000&nfstatusdescription=ERROR%3a+No+local+token.

181 In a phase 1 study of a peanut vaccine called PVX108: Boyles SW. Novel injected peanut allergy treatment shows promise. https://www.medpagetoday.com/meetingcoverage/aaaai/78210.

181 the vaccine did not trigger allergic reactions: Prickett SR, Hickey PLC, Bingham J, et al. Safety and tolerability of a novel peptide-based immunotherapy for peanut allergy. *J Allergy Clin Immunol.* 143(2):AB431.

181 Basophil cells . . . did not become activated in the presence of PVX108: Pharmaceutical Technology. Aravax takes a step closer to developing a peanut allergy vaccine. https://www.pharmaceutical-technology.com/comment/aravax-takes-a-step-closer-to-developing-a-peanut-allergy-vaccine/.

181 Another peanut vaccine, HAL-MPE1: Bindslev-Jensen C, de Kam P-J, van Twuijver E, et al. SCIT-treatment with a chemically modified, aluminum hydroxide adsorbed peanut extract (HAL-MPE1) was generally safe and well tolerated and showed immunological changes in peanut allergic patients. *J Allergy Clin Immunol.* 139(2):AB191.

Chapter 8. Immunotherapy and You

186 In early 2017, two pediatric allergists at Johns Hopkins University: Dunlop JH, Keet CA. Goals and motivations of families pursuing oral immunotherapy for food allergy. *J Allergy Clin Immunol Pract.* 2019;7(2):662–63.e618.

193–94 That's about 18 percent of the country's entire gross domestic product: Centers for Medicare and Medicaid Services. Historical. https://www .cms.gov/Research-Statistics-Data-and-Systems/Statistics-Trends-and-Reports /NationalHealthExpendData/NationalHealthAccountsHistorical.

196 As immunotherapy drugs gain FDA approval, we will learn more about their price tags: Taylor P. Aimmune gets FDA panel backing for peanut allergy therapy. http://www.pmlive.com/pharma_news/aimmune_gets_fda_panel _backing_for_peanut_allergy_therapy_1301656.

196 According to the WHO's interpretation, a drug is cost effective: Institute for Clinical and Economic Review. Evaluating the value of new drugs. http://icer-review.org/wp-content/uploads/2014/01/ICER-value-assessment -framework-for-drug-assessment-and-pricing-reports-v7-26.pdf.

196 An ICER report from June 2019 noted that AR101: Institute for Clinical and Economic Review. A look at oral immunotherapy and Viaskin peanut for peanut allergy. https://icer-review.org/wp-content/uploads/2019/07 /ICER_PeanutAllergy_RAAG_071019.pdf.

197 41 percent of people who are eligible for AR101 could receive the treatment: Institute for Clinical and Economic Review. A look at oral immunotherapy and Viaskin peanut for peanut allergy. https://icer-review.org/wp-content/uploads/2019/07/ICER_PeanutAllergy _RAAG_071019.pdf.

197 That position was flawed: Eiwegger T, Anagnostou K, Arasi S, et al. ICER report for peanut OIT comes up short. *Ann Allergy Asthma Immunol.* 2019;123(5):430–32.

197 A study of epicutaneous peanut immunotherapy and oral peanut immunotherapy: Shaker M, Greenhawt M. Estimation of health and economic benefits of commercial peanut immunotherapy products: A cost-effectiveness analysis. *JAMA Netw Open.* 2019;2(5):e193242.

198 The cellular mechanisms that once made the body break out in hives: Moran TP, Burks AW. Is clinical tolerance possible after allergen immunotherapy? *Curr Allergy Asthma Rep.* 2015;15(5):23.

Chapter 9. The (Not-Too-Distant) Future of Food Allergy Care

211 pulsing peanuts with ultraviolet light: Khamsi R. Is it possible to make a less allergenic peanut? https://www.nytimes.com/2016/12/15/magazine/is -it-possible-to-make-a-less-allergenic-peanut.html.

211 These proteins—Ara h1, Ara h2, Ara h3, and Ara h6: Koppelman SJ, Wensing M, Ertmann M, et al. Relevance of Ara h1, Ara h2 and Ara h3 in peanut-allergic patients, as determined by immunoglobulin E Western blotting, basophil-histamine release and intracutaneous testing: Ara h2 is the most important peanut allergen. *Clin Exp Allergy.* 2004;34(4):583–90; Joost S, Maarten P, Geert H, et al. The individual role of peanut proteins Ara h1, 2, 3, and 6 in peanut allergy. *Clin Transl Allergy.* 2011;1.

211 Researchers then at North Carolina Agricultural and Technical State University created an enzyme solution: Food Safety News. Hypoallergenic peanuts move closer to commercial reality. https://www.foodsafetynews.com/2014/06/hypoallergenic-peanut-products -one-step-closer-to-commercial-reality/#more-92889.

211 Skin prick tests conducted with the altered legumes: Sullivan G. Researchers say they have invented a non-allergenic peanut. https://www .washingtonpost.com/news/morning-mix/wp/2014/08/27/researchers-say-they -have-invented-non-allergenic-peanuts/; Food Safety News. Hypoallergenic peanuts move closer to commercial reality. https://www.foodsafetynews.com /2014/06/hypoallergenic-peanut-products-one-step-closer-to-commercial-reality /#more-92889.

211 A team in Alabama has tried eliminating the gene encoding Ara h2: Dodo HW, Konan KN, Chen FC, et al. Alleviating peanut allergy using genetic engineering: The silencing of the immunodominant allergen Ara h2 leads to its significant reduction and a decrease in peanut allergenicity. *Plant Biotechnol J.* 2008;6(2):135–45.

211 The technology enables scientists to alter genes both inexpensively and easily: Bennett J. 11 crazy gene-hacking things we can do with CRISPR. https://www.popularmechanics.com/science/a19067/11-crazy-things-we-can -do-with-crispr-cas9/.

211 With their identity thus altered, the immune system would no longer attack them: Lewis T. In five years, we could be eating a new kind of GMO. https://www.businessinsider.com/crispr-allergy-free-gmo-peanuts -2015-10.

211 Peggy Ozias-Akins, a molecular geneticist at the University of Georgia: Splitter J. Allergy-free peanuts? Not so fast. https://blogs.scientificamerican.com/guest-blog/allergy-free-peanuts -not-so-fast/.

211–12 Removing all the genes responsible for all the allergenic proteins . . . in the peanut genome: Khamsi R. Is it possible to make a less allergenic peanut? https://www.nytimes.com/2016/12/15/magazine/is-it-possible -to-make-a-less-allergenic-peanut.html.

212 The peanut genome was fully sequenced in 2019: Science Daily. Researchers crack the peanut genome. https://www.sciencedaily.com/releases /2019/05/190502143351.htm.

212 Hortense Dodo at the University of Alabama: Dodo HW, Arntzen CJ, Viquez OM, Konan KNd. Down-regulation and silencing of allergen genes in transgenic peanut seeds. https://patents.google.com/patent/US8217228.

212 In 2018, she described her genetically engineered peanut plant: McRobbie LR. Allergies change how we all eat. http://apps.bostonglobe.com /ideas/graphics/2018/11/the-next-bite/the-ingredients/.

212 the food industry could use her modified peanut: Ibid.

212 eliminated allergenic protein from peanut plants through breeding: Perkins T, Schmitt DA, Isleib TG, et al. Breeding a hypoallergenic peanut. *J Allergy Clin Immunol.* 2008;117(2):S328.

213 make the immune system forget that it ever recognized a food protein as an enemy: Al-Kouba J, Wilkinson AN, Starkey MR, et al. Allergen-encoding bone marrow transfer inactivates allergic T cell responses, alleviating airway inflammation. *JCI Insight.* 2017;2(11).

213 The researchers, led by immunologist Ray Steptoe: Science Daily. Gene therapy could "turn off" severe allergies. https://www.sciencedaily.com /releases/2017/06/170602090731.htm; Al-Kouba J, Wilkinson AN, Starkey MR, et al. Allergen-encoding bone marrow transfer inactivates allergic T cell responses, alleviating airway inflammation. *JCI Insight.* 2017;2(11).

214 the Food Allergy Science Initiative at the Broad Institute: Synthego. CRISPR could uncover the causes of food allergies. https://www.synthego.com /blog/crispr-could-uncover-the-causes-of-food-allergies.

215 One company is creating a nasal spray form of epinephrine: Bryn Pharma. Program Development. https://brynpharma.com/program.html.

215 the FDA granted the product "fast track designation": Bryn Pharma. Bryn pharma completes dosing in pivotal clinical trial designed to support U.S. approval of intranasal epinephrine spray. https://bryn-api.fishawack.solutions /wp-content/uploads/2019/10/Bryn-Pharma-Corporate-Press-Release-Oct-10.pdf.

216 Aibi is a bracelet that senses changes in histamine levels: Made By Chip studio. AIBI: Anaphylaxis Prevention System for Children. http://madebychip.com/aibi.html; Nguyen M. Wearable allergens-detecting devices. https://www.wearable-technologies.com/2016/09/wearable-allergens-detecting -devices/.

216 An accompanying device would deliver epinephrine automatically: Riemer E. Teen's death from allergic reaction inspires work on lifesaving devices. https://www.wcvb.com/article/teens-death-from-allergic-reaction-inspires -work-on-lifesaving-devices/24888841.

216 is named after Abbie Benford, who died from anaphylaxis in 2013: Wyss Institute. Project Abbie. https://wyss.harvard.edu/technology /project-abbie/.

217 According to U.S. regulation, a food must contain less than 20 parts per million (ppm) of gluten: U.S. Food and Drug Administration. "Gluten-free" means what it says. https://www.fda.gov /consumers/consumer-updates/gluten-free-means-what-it-says.

217 In a study published in March 2019, researchers tested the ability of Nima: Zhang J, Portela SB, Horrell JB, et al. An integrated, accurate, rapid, and economical handheld consumer gluten detector. *Food Chem.* 2019;275:446–56.

217 In a 2018 study, the device had a harder time detecting gluten at 20 ppm: Taylor SL, Nordlee JA, Jayasena S, Baumert JL. Evaluation of a handheld gluten detection device. *J Food Prot.* 2018;81(10):1723–28.

217 As journalist Alex Shultz explained in a thorough review of Nima: Shultz A. The potentially perilous promise of food allergen sensors. https://www.theverge.com/2019/4/1/18080666/nima-sensor-testing-fda -food-allergy-gluten-peanut-transparency-data.

218 Two outside tests of the peanut sensor were conducted: Shultz A. The potentially perilous promise of food allergen sensors. https://www .theverge.com/2019/4/1/18080666/nima-sensor-testing-fda-food-allergy-gluten -peanut-transparency-data.

219 There is no established standard for peanut equivalent to the 20 ppm considered safe for gluten: Ibid.

219 The group reported the initial success of their invention in the journal *ACS Nano* in 2017: American Association for the Advancement of Science (AAAS). Keychain detector could catch food allergens before it's too late. https://www.eurekalert.org/pub_releases/2017-09/acs-kdc090617.php; Lin HY, Huang CH, Park J, et al. Integrated magneto-chemical sensor for on-site food allergen detection. *ACS Nano.* 2017;11(10):10062–69.

219 an allergen extraction kit: McDermott B. Meet iEAT: This pocket-sized food allergen detector could save your life. https://www.ireviews.com/news /2017/09/12/ieat-allergen-detector.

219 The group tested five allergens: Lin HY, Huang CH, Park J, et al. Integrated magneto-chemical sensor for on-site food allergen detection. *ACS Nano.* 2017;11(10):10062–69.

220 The device is not yet commercially available: Cox S. Made in Brunel: A portable food allergen test designed to check 'free-from' meals. https://www .brunel.ac.uk/news-and-events/news/articles/Made-in-Brunel-Portable-food -allergen-test-designed-to-check-%27free-from%27-meals.

220 an immediate alert on the keychain device: Allergy Amulet. The science behind our sensors: Molecular Detection. https://www.allergyamulet .com/technology.

221 Within a few seconds, the cloud sends back a list: Tellspec. Tellspec's Mission. http://tellspec.com/faq/#toggle-id-1.

221 And the data from the scan is saved in the cloud: YouTube. Making food transparent | Isabel Hoffmann. https://www.youtube.com /watch?v=nk9dO6XOjrc&feature=youtu.be.

221 One of the lead developers behind Tellspec, Isabel Hoffmann: Ibid.

222 A similar device, SCiO, is a mini sensor: SCiO by Consumer Physics. https://shop.consumerphysics.com.

222 as few as four shots of vaccine: Drug Development and Delivery. DNA vaccine technology—a vaccine breakthrough that could change lives & enable vaccine development programs. https://drug-dev.com /dna-vaccine-technology-a-vaccine-breakthrough-that-could-change-lives-enable -vaccine-development-programs/.

223 ARA-LAMP-Vax could be effective in treating peanut allergy: Li X-M, Song Y, Su Y, et al. Immunization with ARA h1,2,3-Lamp-Vax peanut vaccine blocked IgE mediated-anaphylaxis in a peanut allergic murine model. *J Allergy Clin Immunol.* 2015;135(2):AB167.

223 A phase 1 study, funded by grant money and the drugmaker: ClinicalTrials.gov. A Study to Evaluate Safety, Tolerability and Immune Response in Adults Allergic to Peanut After Receiving Intradermal or Intramuscular Administration of ASP0892 (ARA-LAMP-vax), a Single Multivalent Peanut (Ara h1, h2, h3) Lysosomal Associated Membrane Protein DNA Plasmid Vaccine. https://clinicaltrials.gov/ct2/show /NCT02851277.

223 Another vaccine, PVX108, developed by Robyn O'Hehir and her colleagues in Australia: Pharmaceutical Technology. Aravax takes a step closer to developing a peanut allergy vaccine. https://www.pharmaceutical -technology.com/comment/aravax-takes-a-step-closer-to-developing-a-peanut -allergy-vaccine/.

223 a segment of the genetic sequence from the monoclonal antibody used in omalizumab: Crystal R. New gene therapy protects against peanut allergy. https://news.weill.cornell.edu.

223 When they injected that virus into peanut-allergic mice: Pagovich OE, Wang B, Chiuchiolo MJ, et al. Anti-hIgE gene therapy of peanut-induced anaphylaxis in a humanized murine model of peanut allergy. *J Allergy Clin Immunol.* 2016;138(6):1652–62, e1657.

224 many creative approaches to treatment: Chen M, Land M. The current state of food allergy therapeutics. *Hum Vaccin Immunother.* 2017;13(10): 2434–42.

224 dendritic cells can field multiple allergens at once: Sampath V, Nadeau KC. Newly identified T cell subsets in mechanistic studies of food immunotherapy. *J Clin Invest.* 2019;129(4):1431–40.

224 In a recent study at Stanford, we randomized 20 adults with severe peanut allergy to either an antibody that inhibits IL-33 or a

placebo. Chinthrajah S, Cao S, Liu C, et al. Phase 2a randomized, placebo-controlled study of anti-IL-33 in peanut allergy. *JCI Insight.* 2019;4(22).

225 A long list of experimental drugs: Bauer RN, Manohar M, Singh AM, et al. The future of biologics: applications for food allergy. *J Allergy Clin Immunol.* 2015;135(2):312–23.

225–26 Hidden in this way, the protein could escape the initial allergic response: Takeda. Takeda acquires license for first-in-class celiac disease therapy from COUR Pharmaceuticals following positive phase 2a proof-of-concept study. https://www.takeda.com/newsroom/newsreleases/2019/takeda-acquires-license-for-first-in-class-celiac-disease-therapy-from-cour-pharmaceuticals-following-positive-phase-2a-proof-of-concept-study/.

227 None of the infants who completed the mix arm of the study: Spoonful One. Protection possible with food allergy protection plan. http://hcp.spoonfulone.com.

228 tapping the button sends out a message to emergency responders and personal emergency contacts: Hinkel K. Rescufy launches anaphylaxis emergency mobile app. https://www.pci.upenn.edu/pcinews/rescufy-launches-anaphylaxis-emergency-mobile-app/.

228 by 2025, allergy treatment market will represent a $40 billion market: Cision. Allergy treatment market to reach $40.36 bn, globally, by 2025 at 6.3% CAGR, says Allied Market Research. https://www.prnewswire.com/news-releases/allergy-treatment-market-to-reach-40-36-bn-globally-by-2025-at-6-3-cagr-says-allied-market-research-803169902.html.

229 the global peanut allergy market would grow by 90 percent from 2019 to 2023: Cision. The global peanut allergy market is forescasted [*sic*] to grow at a CAGR of 89.68% during the period 2019–2023. https://www.prnewswire.com/news-releases/the-global-peanut-allergy-market-is-forescasted-to-grow-at-a-cagr-of-89-68-during-the-period-2019-2023–300749510.html.

Chapter 10. The Emotional Toll of Food Allergy

235 A group of pediatric allergists and psychologists from the University of Maryland asked 87 caregivers: Bollinger ME, Dahlquist LM, Mudd K, et al. The impact of food allergy on the daily activities of children and their families. *Ann Allergy Asthma Immunol.* 2006;96:415–21.

235 A group of researchers in the UK: Avery NJ, King RM, Knight S, Hourihane, JO. Assessment of quality of life in children with peanut allergy. *Pediatr Allergy Immunol.* 2003;14:378–82.

236 If young adults with food allergy are self-conscious: Lyons AC, Forde EME. Food allergy in young adults: perceptions and psychological effects. *J Health Psychol.* 2004;9.

236 A study from many years ago found that most teens: Gowland MH. Food allergen avoidance—the patient's viewpoint. *Allergy.* 2001;56 Suppl 67:117–120.

236 Researchers in New Zealand asked a group of young adults: Lyons AC, Forde EME. Food allergy in young adults: perceptions and psychological effects. *J Health Psychol.* 2004;9.

237 It can be tricky, a group of pediatricians wrote: Herbert L, Shemesh E, Bender B. Clinical management of psychosocial concerns related to food allergy. *J Allergy Clin Immunol.* 2016;4:205–13.

239 In 2017, a dairy-allergic British teenager died: Siddique H. Boy with allergy died after cheese was flicked at him, inquest told. *The Guardian.* May 2, 2019.

239 80 of the 251 children surveyed said they'd been bullied: Annunziato RA, Rubes M, Ambrose MA, et al. Longitudinal evaluation of food allergy–related bullying. *J Allergy Clin Immunol.* 2014;2: 639–41.

239 three quarters of the children who'd been bullied a year earlier: Ibid.

239 two thirds of 174 food-allergic teenagers: Sampson MA, Muñoz-Furlong A, Sicherer SH. Risk-taking and coping strategies of adolescents and young adults with food allergy. *J Allergy Clin Immunol.* 2006;117: 1440–45.

240 mothers, the study found, report their teens: Ferro MA, Van Lieshout RJ, Ohayon J, Scott JG. Emotional and behavioral problems in adolescents and young adults with food allergy. *Allergy.* 2016;71:532–40.

240 teens were under-reporting or the moms were over-reporting: Science Daily. It's Mom who sees troubles for teens with food allergies. January 20, 2016.

241 Psychologists have identified several personality traits: Conner TS, Mirosa M, Bremer P, Peniamina R. The role of personality in daily food allergy experiences. *Front Psychol.* 6 Febr 2018. https://www.frontiersin.org /articles/10.3389/fpsyg.2018.00029/full.

242 But it's good to know the signs of anxiety overload: Herzog J. Managing the emotional impact of living with a food allergy. Webinar presented by Food Allergy Research and Education (FARE).

253 the children in this group had fewer mild symptoms as the OIT dose increased: Howe LC, Leibowitz KA, Perry MA, et al. Changing mindsets about non-life-threatening symptoms during oral immunotherapy: a randomized clinical trial. *J Allergy Clin Immunol.* 2019;7:1550–59.

Chapter 11. The Future of the End of Food Allergy

258 adopting a "Westernized" lifestyle may be contributing to food allergy diagnoses: Prescott SL, Pawanker R, Allen KJ, et al. A global survey of changing patterns of food allergy burden in children. *World Allergy Org J.* 2013;6:1–12.

258 the extent of the condition across the continent: Burney PG, Potts J, Kummeling I, Mills EN. The prevalence and distribution of food sensitization in European adults. *Allergy.* 2014:69:365–71.

259 Slovenia, Estonia, Switzerland, Greece, and Belgium: Steinke M, Fiocchi A, Kirchlechner V, et al. Perceived food allergy in children in 10 European nations. A randomised telephone survey. *Int Arch Allergy Immunol.* 2007;143:290–95.

259 3 percent of 1-year-olds and more than 7 percent of 8-year-olds: Ostblom E, Lilja G, Pershagen G, et al. Phenotypes of food hypersensitivity and development of allergic diseases during the first 8 years of life. *Clin Exp Allergy.* 2008;38:1325–32.

260 Studies in Ghana: Obeng BB, Amoah AS, Larbi IA, et al. Food allergy in Ghanaian schoolchildren: data on sensitization and reported food allergy. *Int Arch Allergy Immunol.* 2011;155:63–73.

260 and South Africa: Levin ME, Le Souëf PN, Motala C. Total IgE in urban Black South African teenagers: the influence of atopy and helminth infection. *Pediatr Allergy Immunol.* 2008;19:449–54.

260 400 households in Tanzania: Justin-Temu M, Risha P, Abla O, Massawe A. Incidence, knowledge and health seeking behavior for perceived allergies at household level: a case study in Ilala district Dar es Salaam Tanzania. *East Afr J Public Health.* 2008;5:90–93.

260 a 2005 study in Mozambique: Lunet N, Falcão H, Sousa M et al. Self-reported food and drug allergy in Maputo, Mozambique. *Public Health.* 2005;119:587–89.

260 China has been paying attention: Prescott SL, Pawanker R, Allen KJ, et al. A global survey of changing patterns of food allergy. *World Allergy Org J.* 2013;6:1–12.

260 more than 30,000 people in Taiwan: Wu TC, Tsai TC, Huang CF, et al. Prevalence of food allergy in Taiwan: a questionnaire-based survey. *Intern Med J.* 2012;42:1310–15.

260 A study in South India: Mahesh PA, Wong GW, Ogorodova L, et al. Prevalence of food sensitization and probably food allergy among adults in India: the EuroPrevail INCO Study. *Allergy.* 2016;71:1010–19.

261 Fruit and vegetable allergies are common in Colombia: Marrugo J, Hernández L, Villalba V. Prevalence of self-reported food allergy in Cartagena (Colombia) population. *Allergol Immunopathol (Madr).* 2008;36:320–24.

261 280 out of 2,848 12-month-olds had a bona fide food allergy: Osborne NJ, Koplin JJ, Martin PE, et al. Prevalence of challenge-proven IgE-mediated food allergy using population-based sampling and predetermined challenge criteria in infants. *J Allergy Clin Immunol.* 2011;127:668–76.

261 "food allergy capital of the world": Reddiex S, Nguyen-Robertson C. Why is Australia the food allergy capital of the world? The Royal Society of Victoria. June 18, 2018. https://rsv.org.au/food-allergy-capital/.

261 more common among Arab children: Graif Y, German L, Livne I, Shohat T. Association of food allergy with asthma severity and atopic diseases in Jewish and Arab adolescents. *Acta Paediatr.* 2012;101:1083–88.

261 89-country study: Prescott SL, Pawanker R, Allen KJ, et al. A global survey of changing patterns of food allergy. *World Allergy Org J.* 2013;6:1–12.

262 food allergy already costs an estimated $25 billion per year in just the United States alone: Gupta R, Holdford D, Bilaver L, et al. The economic impact of childhood food allergy in the United States. *JAMA Pediatr.* 2013;167:1026–31.

262 will allow plants to adapt to climate change: Beggs PJ, Walczyk NE. Impacts of climate change on plant food allergens: a previously unrecognized threat to human health. *Air Qual Atmos Health.* 2008;1(2):119–123.

262 amount of allergenic proteins can vary widely: Sampson HA. Update on food allergy. *J Allergy Clin Immunol.* 2004;113(5):805–19.

263 they produced greater concentrations of Ara h1: Ziska LH, Yang J, Tomacek MB, Beggs PJ. Cultivar-specific changes in peanut yield, biomass, and allergenicity in response to elevated atmospheric carbon dioxide concentration. *Crop Science.* 2016;56:2766–74.

263 Pollen records from seventeen different locations in twelve countries: Knowlton K. It's official: climate change worsens pollen season. National Resources Defense Council. March 26, 2019. https://www.nrdc.org/experts/kim-knowlton/its-official-climate-change-worsens-global-pollen-season.

264 regional differences in food allergy caused by oral allergy syndrome: Katelaris CH, Beggs PJ. Climate change: allergens and allergic diseases. *Intern Med J.* 2018;48:129–34.

264 They can also make plants more allergenic: Shahali Y, Dadar M. Plant food allergy: influence of chemicals on plant allergens. *Food Chem Toxicol.* 2018;115:365–74.

265 Reports have linked proteases to dry skin and eczema: Sarlo K, Ritz HL, Fletcher ER, et al. Proteolytic detergent enzymes enhance the allergic antibody responses of guinea pigs to nonproteolytic detergent enzymes in a mixture: Implications for occupational exposure. *J Allergy Clin Immunol.* 1997;100:480–87.

265 mostly from animal studies: Basketter DA, English JS, Wakelin SH, White IR. Enzymes, detergents and skin: facts and fantasies. *Br J Dermatol.* 2008;158:1177–81.

265 detergents can cause skin cells to break apart: Wang M, Tan G, Eljaszewicz A, et al. Laundry detergents and detergent residue after rinsing directly disrupt tight junction barrier integrity in human bronchial epithelial cells. *J Allergy Clin Immunol.* 2019;143:1892–903.

267 Infants and children who maintain skin barrier protection: Nadeau KC, Sindher S, Berdyshev E, et al. Skin TEWL measurements show significant improvement with Trilipid emollient compared to controls in infants and young children. Presented at the annual meeting of the American Academy of Asthma, *Allergy and Immunology.* March 13–16, 2020, Philadelphia, PA.

INDEX

Page numbers in *italics* refer to charts and graphs.

antibodies, 37. *See also*
  immunoglobulin E
antihistamines, 80, 91–92, 112
anxiety
  experienced with immunotherapy,
    233–34, 244–46, 252–53, 254
  helping others cope with, 246–50
  recognizing, 242–44
  See also emotional toll of food
    allergy
apple allergy, 259, *264*
apps, smartphone, 228
apricot allergy, *264*
ARA-LAMP-Vax, 222–23, *226*
AR101 (Palforzia), 112, 157–58, *165,
  166*, 194, 196–97
Asia, prevalence of food allergies in,
  258, 260
asthma
  and atopic march, 31, *32*
  and cesarean sections, 57, 60
  desensitization therapy for, 151
  and epinephrine, 80–81
  and genetics, 46–47, *50*
  and hygiene hypothesis, 23, 25, 26
  and IgE production, 37
  and maternal diet, 51, 53
  and risk of fatal reactions, 85
  role of race/ethnicity in, 20
  and sibling effect, 25
  and Traditional Chinese
    Medicine, 94
  and vitamin D deficiency, 34
atopic dermatitis. *See* eczema
atopic diseases, 31
atopic march, 30–31, *32*, 37, 65, 261
Australia
  clinical trials in, 201
  food labeling regulations in, 79
  prevalence of food allergies in, 20,
    45, 261
  and research on cesarean
    sections, 58
  and research on early egg
    exposure, 135–36, *137, 138*
  and research on emotional/
    behavioral issues of food-allergic
    teens, 240
  and research on infant formula, 55

and research on probiotics, 178
and school policies, 93
sunlight exposure in, 34
Australisian Society of Clinical
  Immunology and Allergy
  (ASCIA), 55, 140, 180
Austria, 26, 201
autoimmune diseases, 149
AUVI-Q (epinephrine injector), 91
avoidance of allergens
  and benefits of early exposure, 113
  choosing, 206
  failure to eliminate food allergies,
    108, 125, 126, 127
  and historical perspectives on food
    allergies, 105–10
  and Learning Early About Peanut
    Allergy (LEAP) trial, 131
  limitations of approach, 150, 202
  and Prevention of Egg Allergy with
    Tiny Amounts (PETIT)
    study, 135
  and prevention of food allergies,
    106–8
  scientific scrutiny of, 108–11
avoidant restrictive food disorder,
  250–51
Avon Longitudinal Study of Parents
  and Children, 52

Bacteroides, 59–60, 61
bananas, *264*
Barnett, Sloan, 10–11, 190–91,
  245, 280
Barnett, Violet, 190–91, 245–46
basophil activation tests (BATs), *119*,
  122–23, 124
basophils, *38*, 122, 181
Beating Egg Allergy Trial (BEAT),
  136, *137*
Before Brands, 227
behavioral issues of food allergic
  teens, 240
Belgium, 259
bell peppers, *264*
Benadryl (diphenhydramine), 92
Benford, Abbie, 216

consciousness, loss of, 86
Consortium of Food Allergy Research (CoFAR), 176
cooking protocols, 69–70
coriander, *264*
corn allergy, 21
cosmetics, 72
costs of immunotherapy, 193–97
coughing, 86, 140
cramps, *83*
creams, 72
CRISPR/Cas9, 211, 212, 214, 229
Crohn's disease, 23, 42
cross-contact/cross-contamination, 70–72, 77, 192
crustacean shellfish allergy, 20, 78
Crystal, Ronald, 223
cucumbers, *264*
Cuellar, Hector, 67–68
Cuellar, Leah, 67–68, 177–78
Cuellar, William, 67–68, 177–78
"cures" for food allergy, 199–200
cytokines, 37

daily life with food allergies, 92–93
dairy allergy, 20, 65, 68, 107, 108.
    See also milk and milk allergies
dairy sensitivity, 41
day care, 25
deaths caused by food allergies, 83–84, 95, 105, 112, 236
delayed exposure to food, 106–11, 113–14, 118, 129–32, 148, 150.
    See also avoidance of allergens
Democritus, 100
Denmark, 58, 201
desensitization, 14, 103–4, 148, 150–51, 152, 198–99. *See also* oral immunotherapy (OIT)
detergents, 265–66
diabetes, 23, 25
DIABIMMUNE study of Broad Institute, 29–30
diagnosis of food allergies
    and basophil activation test, 122–23, 124
    blood tests for, 112, 118–19, 124

and elimination diet, 104
and food diaries, 117, 124
and intradermal test, *119*, 120
and medical history, 115–17
and oral food challenge, 120–22, 124, 130
and scratch test, 111
and skin patch test, *119*, 120
and skin prick test, 102–4, 111, 115, 117–18, 124
dining table, managing cross-contact risks at, 72
diphenhydramine (Benadryl), 92
dirt, exposure to, 23, 30
diversity in diet, 54, 142, 266
dizziness, *83*
DNA LAMP vaccine, *184*
doctors, questions to ask, 203–4
dogs, benefits of, 266
double-blind, placebo-controlled food challenge (DBPCFC), 120–21
dry skin, 23, 31, 148, 267
dual-allergen exposure theory, 31–33
Dunn Galvin, A., *174*
dupilumab (anti-IL-4R), *183*, 200, *225*, 225
Dupont, C., *169*
dust-mite allergens, 110, 111
Du Toit, George, 52, 127

early introduction to allergens, 125–44
    and allergy-preventing treats, 227–28
    to eggs, 135–36, *137–38*
    guidelines for, 133–34, 139–42, 143–44
    and importance of diversity in diet, 142
    and Israel's low incidence of peanut allergy, 127–29
    to multiple allergenic foods, 133, *139*
    to peanuts, 127–33, *139*
    studies on, 129–33, *137–39*
East Asia, 47
Eastern Europe, 59

historical perspectives on food
allergies, 99–112
in ancient times, 100–101
and avoidance paradigm, 105–10
coining of term *allergy*, 101–2, 111
and deaths related to peanut
allergy, 105, 112
and desensitization, 103–4
and division in field of allergy
specialists, 105
and elimination diet, 104, 111
and Schofield's treatment of egg
allergy, 99–100, 111
and skin prick testing, 102–4, 111
timeline of, 111–12
hives, *83*, 84, 91
Hofmann, A. M., *161*
home, reducing allergen risks in
allergens in ingredient lists, 72
cooking protocols, 69–70
cross-contact, 70–72
food labels, 73–79, 95
in the pantry and refrigerator,
68–69, 71
questions to consider, 73
H1 blockers, *83*
honeydews, *264*
Hong Kong, 22, 260
hospital visits related to food
allergies, 20
Hsiao, K. C., *165*
H2 blockers, *83*
human leukocyte antigen (HLA)
system, 48
hygiene hypothesis, 22–28, 29–30,
148, 267
hypoallergenic term in food
labeling, 78
hypotension, *83*, 86

ice, application of, *83*, 92
Iceland, 20, 201
identity, influence of food allergy
on, 244
iEAT food sensor, 219–20
IgE-ImmunoCAP test, *119*
IgE-mediated allergy, 14, 35–36

IgE to components test, *119*
IgG4 antibodies, 120, 131, 149,
177, 253
immune system
and avoidance paradigm, 113
and food intolerance vs. allergy, 43
and gene therapy, 213
and hygiene hypothesis, 23–28
and science behind food allergy,
35–40, *38*
Immune Tolerance Network, 214
immunoglobulin E (IgE)
about, 14
and avoidance diet/paradigm,
106, 131
and celiac disease, 278
and cesarean sections, 58–59
and chain of immune response,
36–37, *38*, 39, 43, 148
and changes to allergenic
foods, 263
and clinical trials for oral
immunotherapy, 159
discovery of, 36, 112
and drugs under investigation,
225, *225*
and early exposure to
allergens, 131
and epicutaneous
immunotherapy, 177
and food intolerance vs. allergy,
14, 43
and food labeling regulations, 78
function of, 148
and genetically altered foods, 211
and genetics, 38–39
high levels of, 193
IgG4 antibodies' ability to
block, 149
and immunotherapy, 148–49,
152–53, 185
and maternal diet, 52
and omalizumab, 160, 223
as reliable indicator of food allergy,
106, 148
and science behind food allergy,
35–40, *38*
and testing, 115, 117, 118, *119*, 120,
122, 124

immunotherapy (IT)
about, 4, 5, 146, 147–49
anxiety experienced with, 244–46, 252–53, 254
basic principle underlying, 148–49
cautions on attempting at-home treatment, 207–8
and clinical trials, 8, 147
costs of, 193–97
delaying, 206
epicutaneous (EPIT), 112, *169*, 176–78, 179, *184*, 194, 197
history of research on, 150–56
at private clinics, 204–5
and probiotics, 178–79
public perception of, 187, 207
questions to consider in, 203–4
subcutaneous (SCIT), 112, 151, *183*
sublingual (SLIT), 175–76, 179, *183*
See also oral immunotherapy (OIT)
India, 260
inflammation, 37
inflammatory bowel disease, 42, 60, 61
influenza vaccines, 79
ingredient sensors, 216–22
Institute for Clinical and Economic Review (ICER), 196–97
intolerance, 14
intradermal test, *119*, 120
IPEX syndrome, *50*
Ireland, 57, 201
Ishizaka, Kimishige, 36
Ishizaka, Teruko, 36
Isle of Wight, 47, 110
Israel, 127–29, 131, 156, 171, 201, 261
Israel Association of Allergy and Clinical Immunology, 126
Italy, 25, 259
itching, *83*, 84, 91

Japan, 135, *137*, 155, *165*, 260
Johansson, Gunnar, 36
Johns Hopkins University, 154, 176, 186

Jones, S., 156, *161*, *170*
Jung, Scott, 189–90

Katz, Yitzhak, 127
kitchen, managing allergen risks in, 68–72
kiwi allergy, 259, *264*
Korea, 260
kosher foods, 76
Kukkonen, A. K., *164*

Lack, Gideon, 52, 125–33
Lactobacillus rhamnosus, 178
lactose intolerance, 14
LAMP DNA, 181, 222–23
LAMP-Vax, 222–23, *226*
Lancet, The, 57, 100
language of food allergy, 14–15
latex allergy, 41
Learning Early About Peanut Allergy (LEAP and LEAP-ON) trials, 129–33, 135, *139*
legumes, guidelines for introducing, 142. *See also* peanuts and peanut allergy; soy and soy allergy
lethargy, 140
Li, Xiu-Min, 94
lifestyle changes, environmentally friendly, 265–67
light-headedness, 86
Liptak, Amelia, 90
Liptak, Elizabeth, 90
Lithuania, 259
loratadine (Claritin), *83*, 91
lotions, 72
low birth weight, 65

MacGinnitie, A. J., *164*
Maimonides, Moses, 101, 111
maintenance doses, 172, 198, 208
mast cells, 37, *38*, 39, 112

National Health and Nutrition
Examination Survey
(NHANES), 17–18, 34
National Institute of Allergy
and Infectious Diseases
(NIAID), 110, 112, 133–34,
140, 200
National Institutes of Health (NIH),
201, 214
nature and outdoors, time in, 267
Netherlands, the, 26–27, 33,
60, 201
*New England Journal of Medicine,
The*, 132, 157
New Zealand, 79
nickle allergy, 126
Nima ingredient sensors, 216–18
North Carolina Agricultural and
Technical State University,
211, 212
Northwestern University, 227
nose congestion or itchiness, 91
Nowak-Wegrzyn, Anna,
29, *170*
nucleotide polymorphisms (SNPs),
48–49
nut allergies
and allergen-free tables in school
cafeterias, 93
and foods packaged at facilities
processing nuts, 192–93
and genetics, *49*
and managing risks in the home,
68–69
and oral food challenge, 121
See also peanuts and peanut
allergy; tree nuts and tree nut
allergies
Nutrition Labeling and Education
Act, 74

oats and oat allergy, 33, 40
obesity, 61, 62
O'Hehir, Robyn, 223
oils, food-based, 72, 77–78
"old friends" theory, 28–31
Oliver, George, 81

omalizumab in combination with
oral immunotherapy
administration of, 192
and Barnett's IT treatment, 245
benefits of, 193
clinical trials involving, 8, 160–61,
162, 164, 168, *169, 173, 183*, 200
function of, 160
limitations of, 223
summary of research results, *182*
and timeline of food allergy
research, 112
onions, *264*
oral allergy syndrome, 40–41
oral food challenge, 120–22, 124,
130, 153, 190–91, 258
oral immunotherapy (OIT)
AAP's guidelines on, 180
about, 146
age of participants in, 189
anti-IL-4R antibody in
combination with, *183*
anxiety experienced with, 252–53
cautions on attempting at-home
treatment, 207–8
clinical trials for, 156–60, *161–67*,
194–95, 200–202, 208
committing to, 188
costs of, 193–97
EAACI's guidelines on, 179
early research on, 151, 152–56
effect on quality of life, 171–72,
173–75
enrolling in studies, 200–202, 208
four steps of, 153
goals of patients in, 191
maintenance doses in, 172, 198, 208
medications in combination with,
160–61. *See also* omalizumab
medicinal application of food in,
153–54
motives for pursuing, 186–88
and oral food challenge, 190–91
probiotics in combination with,
178–79, *182*
public perception of, 187
questions to consider, 203–4
and Schofield's treatment of egg
allergy, 147

summary of research results,
161–67
triggered by birch pollen, *264*
vaccines for, 181, *184*, 223
and vitamin D deficiency, 34
pear allergy, *264*
pecans, *173*
pectin, 72
Pepcid, *83*
peppers, sensitivity to, 41
peptide immunotherapy, 181
Pepto Bismol, *83*
personality and food allergy,
240–42
pesticides, 76
pistachios, 20
plants, diets lacking in, 30
Platt-Mills, Thomas, 41
plum allergy, *264*
policies and practices that impact
food, 268–69
Pollan, Michael, 266
pollen, 40–41, 47, 51, 111,
263–64, *264*
Portugal, 113
potatoes, *264*
prebiotics, 142–43
predisposition to food allergies, 110
pregnancy diet and infant food
allergies, 50–54, 55, *64*, 66,
106–7, 108
premature birth, 65
prevalence of food allergies
in Africa, 260
in Asia, 260
in Australia, 261
and avoidance paradigm, 108
in Europe, 258–59
and history of food allergy
research, 150
in the Middle East, 261
and most common allergens, *21*
rising rates of, 17–22, *18*, *19*, 43,
108, 258
in South America, 261
prevention diet, 106–8
Prevention of Egg Allergy with
Tiny Amounts (PETIT),
135, *137*

private clinics, immunotherapy
at, 204–5
probiotics
combined with immunotherapy,
163, *165*, *174*, 178–79, *182*
inconclusive evidence on, 30–31,
142–43
produce, 76
Protection Against Allergy: Study in
Rural Environments
(PASTURE), 142
Prunicki, Mary, 262
psychosomatic allergy symptoms,
104–5, 242
Puerto Rico, 62
pulse, weak, 86
Pure Food and Drug Act
(Wiley Act), 74
PVX108 vaccine, 181, *184*, 223

quality of life, 171–72, *173–75*,
234–35

race and ethnicity, 20–22
ragweed pollen, *264*
rashes, 14. *See also* skin barrier
rate of food allergies. *See* prevalence
of food allergies
recalls, food, 74
redness, 91
refined oils, 77–78
refrigerator, managing
allergen risks in,
68–69, 71
Reier-Nilson, T., *175*
Rescufy, 228
restaurants, 70–71, 76, 249
rhinitis, *32*
rhinovirus, 27
rice, 40
Richard III, King of England, 101
Rook, Graham, 28
Roosevelt, Theodore, 74
Rowe, Albert, 104, 111
royal jelly allergy, 22

RSV (respiratory syncytial virus), 27
runny nose, *83*
rural and farming communities,
    prevalence of allergies in, 25, 26,
    27, 34–35

vaginal seeding, 62–63
Varshney, P., *162*
Viaskin, 177, *184*
Vickery, B. P., *162*, *164*, *166*
vitamin D deficiency, 33–35, 266–67
vomiting, *83*, 140
Von Pirquet, Clemens, 101–2, 111

walnuts, 20, 47, *173*
watermelons, *264*
wearables, 216
Weill Cornell Medicine, 223
wheat and wheat allergy
    and avoidance paradigm, 127
    and clinical trials for oral
        immunotherapy, *170*
    and food labeling regulations, 79
    and genetics, 47
    guidelines for introducing, 142
    historical perspectives on, 101
    and managing risks in the home,
        69–70

prevalence of, 20, *21*
and race/ethnicity, 21
and sensors that detect
    ingredients, 219
symptoms of, *83*
wheezing, *83*, 88
Wiley Act (Pure Food and Drug
    Act), 74
Wood, Robert, 154
World Allergy Organization, 18, 82
World Health Organization (WHO),
    54, 196
Wu Mei Wan, 94

Yates, Kim, 145, 167–68,
    192, 238, 280

Zantac (ranitidine), *83*
zucchinis, *264*
Zyrtec (cetirizine), *83*, 91